Essentials of Clinical Epilepsy

Essentials of Clinical Epilepsy

Second Edition

Alan H. Guberman, B.Sc., M.D., F.R.C.P.(C)

Professor of Medicine (Neurology), University of Ottawa Faculty of Medicine, Ontario, Canada; Director, Epilepsy Clinic and EEG/Video Intensive Monitoring Laboratory, and Attending Neurologist, Ottawa Hospital, Ontario

J. Bruni, B.Sc., M.D., F.R.C.P.(C)

Associate Professor of Medicine (Neurology), University of Toronto Faculty of Medicine, Ontario, Canada; Consultant Neurologist, St. Michael's Hospital, Toronto

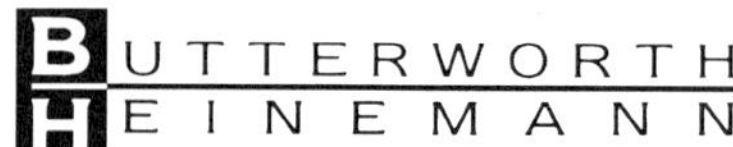

Boston Oxford Auckland Johannesburg Melbourne New Delhi

A member of the Reed Elsevier group

Every effort has been made to ensure that the drug dosage schedules within this text are accurate and conform to standards accepted at time of publication. However, as treatment recommendations vary in the light of continuing research and clinical experience, the reader is advised to verify drug dosage schedules herein with information found on product information sheets. This is especially true in cases of new or infrequently used drugs.

Recognizing the importance of preserving what has been written, Butterworth-Heinemann prints its books on acid-free paper whenever possible.

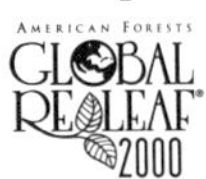

Butterworth-Heinemann supports the efforts of American Forests and the Global ReLeaf program in its campaign for the betterment of trees, forests, and our environment.

Library of Congress Cataloging-in-Publication Data

Guberman, Alan.
Essentials of clinical epilepsy / Alan Guberman, J. Bruni. -- 2nd ed.
p. cm.
Rev. ed. of: Clinical handbook of epilepsy. c1997.
Includes bibliographical references and index.
ISBN 0-7506-7109-2
1. Epilepsy. I. Bruni, J. (Joseph) II. Guberman, Alan. Clinical handbook of epilepsy. III. Title.
[DNLM: 1. Epilepsy. WL 385 G921 1999]
RC372.G73 1999
616.8'53--dc21
DNLM/DLC
for Library of Congress 98-50640
CIP

British Library Cataloguing-in-Publication Data

A catalogue record for this book is available from the British Library.

The publisher offers special discounts on bulk orders of this book.
For information, please contact:

Manager of Special Sales
Butterworth-Heinemann
225 Wildwood Avenue
Woburn, MA 01801-2041
Tel: 781-904-2500
Fax: 781-904-2620

For information on all Butterworth-Heinemann publications available, contact our World Wide Web home page at http://www.bh.com

10 9 8 7 6 5 4 3 2 1

Printed in the United States of America

Contents

About the Authors

Alan H. Guberman, B.Sc., M.D., F.R.C.P.(C), is Professor of Medicine (Neurology) at the University of Ottawa Faculty of Medicine and Director of the Epilepsy Clinic and EEG/Video Intensive Monitoring Laboratory at the Ottawa Hospital, General Site, Ottawa, Ontario, Canada. He trained in the fields of neurology and epilepsy at the McGill University Faculty of Medicine, at the Washington University School of Medicine, and in Marseille, France, at the Centre St.-Paul. For the last 10 years, Dr. Guberman has been actively engaged in clinical trials of new antiepileptic drugs and has published and lectured extensively on epilepsy. Among his publications are three books—*An Introduction to Clinical Neurology*, *Atlas of Electroencephalography*, *Visual Diagnosis: Self Tests in Epilepsy*—and a CD-ROM, *Epilepsy*, published by Corel. Dr. Guberman is a member of the Canadian Neurological Society, the American Academy of Neurology, the American Epilepsy Society, and the Canadian Medical Association. He is also director of the Neurology Residency Program at the University of Ottawa, chairman of the Education Subcommittee of the Canadian League Against Epilepsy, and a past president of the Canadian League Against Epilepsy.

J. Bruni, B.Sc., M.D., F.R.C.P.(C), is Associate Professor of Medicine (Neurology) at the University of Toronto Faculty of Medicine and St. Michael's Hospital, Toronto, Ontario, Canada. He trained in the fields of medicine, neurology, and epilepsy at the McGill University Faculty of Medicine, the University of Toronto Faculty of Medicine, and the University of Florida College of Medicine. With a special interest in epilepsy, Dr. Bruni has done extensive research in the clinical investigation of new antiepileptic drugs. He has published and lectured widely on epilepsy and has been involved in multiple continuing education programs in Canada and the United States. He is a past president of the Canadian League Against Epilepsy and a member of the Canadian Congress of Neurological Sciences, the American Academy of Neurology, the American Epilepsy Society, the Canadian Medical Association, and the Scientific Council of Epilepsy Canada. Dr. Bruni is coauthor of the textbook *Seizure Disorders: A Pharmacological Approach to Treatment* and the CD-ROM *A Clinical Guide to Epileptic Seizures*, as well as editor of the manual *Demystifying Epilepsy*, published by the Canadian Medical Association.

Preface

Epilepsy is an age-old condition, the understanding of which has increased immensely over the past two decades. A clearer grasp of its pathophysiology, the development of advanced neuroimaging techniques, efforts to improve and standardize classification, the advent of new pharmacotherapies with fewer side effects, greater knowledge of pharmacokinetic principles, the application of results from increasingly well-designed clinical trials, and refinements in the surgical therapy of epilepsy have all contributed to the improved welfare of epilepsy patients. These developments have improved patient care and caused a remarkable resurgence of interest in epilepsy among neurologists, neurosurgeons, and neuroscientists. Epilepsy has become one of the most dynamically evolving therapeutic fields in neurology.

This handbook presents the core clinical knowledge on epilepsy in a concise and up-to-date manner. Numerous tables and figures summarize the material, and fairly extensive lists of suggested reading are included. The hope is that residents in neurology; general neurologists; and specialists in fields such as family and internal medicine, emergency medicine, and psychiatry will use this as a quick and convenient reference. Patients and their families may also benefit from consulting this volume, which is not only comprehensive and current but also digestible.

The points of view expressed are strictly those of the authors, and although all drug dosages and therapeutic recommendations have been checked with standard sources, we have presented our own habits and biases in the use of these drugs. We hope that this book will contribute to improving the quality of life of epileptic patients by augmenting the expertise of their caregivers.

A. Guberman
J. Bruni

Acknowledgments

The authors thank Ms. Claire Loyer and Ms. Lorna Mirambel for their assistance in the preparation of the manuscript. We also thank Serge Moraca of Meducom for his valuable suggestions during preparation of the first edition and Carter Snead III, M.D., for his contribution of material on neonatal seizures to the first edition. In addition, we are grateful to Steve Grahovac, M.D., who kindly provided some of the neuroimaging figures for this edition. We also thank Susan Pioli of Butterworth-Heinemann for her support of and useful input to this project, as well as Allison Spearman of Silverchair Science + Communications, who copyedited the book.

Essentials of Clinical Epilepsy

1 Terminology

Epilepsy: A chronic condition of various etiologies characterized by a predisposition to recurrent, usually spontaneous, epileptic seizures.

- A single seizure does not constitute epilepsy. Two initial seizures occurring within a 24-hour period are considered to have the same significance as a single seizure. However, a single seizure accompanied by evidence of a cortical lesion (e.g., abnormalities on neurologic examination, such as mental retardation, or on neuroimaging) or a single seizure accompanied by epileptiform abnormalities on electroencephalography (EEG) could serve as the basis for a diagnosis of epilepsy.
- Reflex epilepsies occur primarily in response to a specific sensory stimulus and are therefore not spontaneous.

Epileptic seizure: An abnormal and excessive discharge of brain neurons involving hypersynchrony accompanied by some behavioral change.

- A seizure may be purely electrical, apparent only on EEG with no obvious clinical manifestation. The symptoms of the seizure may be entirely subjective rather than objective. The behavioral changes accompanying a seizure may be subtle and detectable only by specialized neuropsychological tests such as measurement of reaction time.
- A seizure is not always accompanied by a recordable abnormality on the EEG because it may arise from deep brain structures or may be missed due to spatial sampling errors.

Acute seizures are epileptic seizures resulting from an acute disturbance of brain structure or metabolism or an acute systemic metabolic disturbance. For example, repeated attacks of hypoglycemia, syncope, or ingestion of certain drugs may produce seizures in an individual who is not otherwise predisposed to seizures. The label "epilepsy" is not used because the seizures are closely related to the underlying temporary disturbance of brain function. The term *acute seizures* is used for seizures occurring less than 1–2 weeks after the acute brain or metabolic disturbance.

- Recurrent seizures may occur with metabolic or structural lesions that do not ordinarily produce seizures due to an underlying brain lesion or low genetic threshold for seizures. Such patients could be considered to have epilepsy.

Epilepsy syndrome: A clinical entity with relatively consistent clinical features, including seizure type(s), etiology, EEG features, neurologic status, prognosis, and, in some cases, response to specific antiepileptic drugs.

2 Epidemiology

- After headache, epilepsy is the second most common chronic neurologic condition seen by neurologists.
- The social and personal costs of epilepsy are significant, as evidenced by the high rate of unemployment and underemployment among epileptic patients, and are related to the facts that epilepsy often begins in childhood or early adult life, often is chronic, and has a high prevalence.
- The *prevalence* of epilepsy (proportion of active cases within a particular population at one time) is approximately 1%. Active cases are defined as having had one or more seizures in the previous 5 years. Figures vary according to whether active or inactive cases are considered and according to geographic location (e.g., up to 4–5% in Mexico and certain African countries where cerebral infections, perinatal complications, and head trauma are more common).
- Prevalence is fairly uniform in countries of similar socioeconomic development.
- Prevalence is fairly uniform at different ages, reaching 6–8 cases per 1,000 individuals by adolescence, except for an increase by age 80, when prevalence reaches 23 cases per 100,000 individuals.
- Two percent to 5% of all children experience *febrile seizures* before age 5. *Simple* febrile seizures do *not* carry an increased risk of subsequent epilepsy (see Chapter 3).
- The *incidence of epilepsy* (annual rate of appearance of new cases) is a measure of the number of new cases per 100,000 population per year. It ranges between 40 and 70 per 100,000 in most developed countries and between 100 and 190 per 100,000 in developing countries.
- The age incidence of epilepsy is shown in Figure 2.1. Age peaks of incidence in most countries occur in the first few years of life and in the later years of life, reflecting the multiple etiologies found at the two extremes. Fifty percent to 60% of epilepsy begins before age 16. The age peak in young children has declined, and the peak in the elderly is increasing. In Western countries, the incidence of epilepsy is now higher in people older than age 70 than in people younger than age 10.
- The *cumulative incidence* of epilepsy (chance of acquiring epilepsy at some time during life) is 2–4%. The chances of having *at least one seizure* during a lifetime is approximately 8%. If one includes epilepsy, isolated seizures, acute symptomatic seizures, and febrile seizures, the cumulative incidence is close to 10% by age 80.

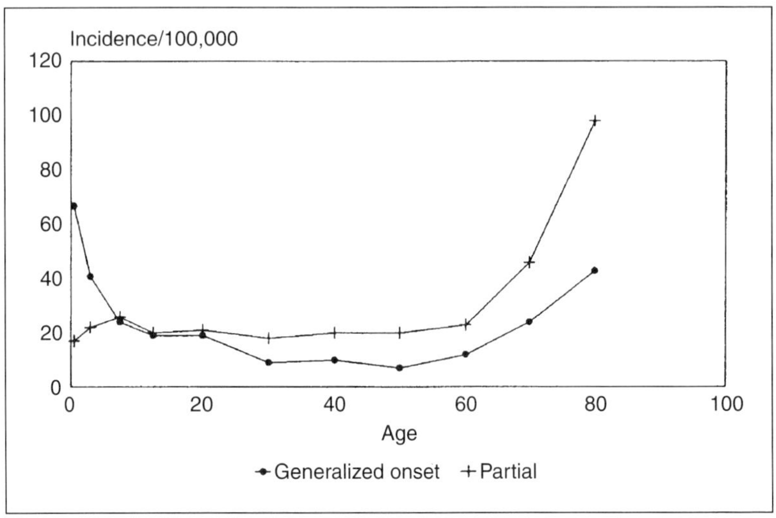

FIGURE 2.1 Age-specific incidence of generalized-onset and partial-onset seizures in Rochester, Minnesota: 1935–1984. (Reprinted with permission from WA Hauser. Seizure disorders: changes with age. Epilepsia 1992;33[Suppl 4]:S9.)

- Of new cases of epilepsy, approximately 50% have seizures of *partial* origin and 50% of *generalized* origin before age 40. After age 40, the proportion of partial epilepsy cases rises to 75% by age 75.
- Epilepsy can be classified etiologically as
  - *Remote symptomatic*: due to a known or identifiable, previously acquired brain lesion.
  - *Cryptogenic*: due to an acquired brain lesion (including prenatally acquired developmental anomalies) that has not been identified or that is of unknown cause. Most partial epilepsies fall into this category.
  - *Idiopathic*: etiology unknown, presumed to be genetic. Most primary generalized epilepsies and benign partial epilepsies of childhood fall into this category.
- Approximately 60% of all epilepsies are idiopathic or cryptogenic.
- Virtually any type of brain pathology can cause seizures/epilepsy, though processes affecting the cerebral cortex are much more likely to do so (see Chapter 3).
- The etiology of seizures is multifactorial in any given individual and is best thought of as an interaction among genetically determined seizure thresholds, underlying predisposing pathologies or metabolic derangements, and acute precipitating factors.

Prognosis of Epilepsy

Prognosis can be discussed in terms of

- Prognosis for long-term seizure remission (treated or untreated)
- Long-term psychosocial outcome
- Morbidity and mortality related to epilepsy

Prognosis for Remission

- A community-based study by Annegers et al. (1979) from the Mayo Clinic showed that approximately 65% of patients achieve a 5-year remission by 10 years after diagnosis and that approximately 75% of patients achieve a 5-year remission by 20 years postdiagnosis. Seventy percent of patients in remission were off medication. Remission was achieved by 85% of patients with generalized tonic-clonic seizures, 80% of patients with absence seizures, and 65% of patients with complex partial seizures. With idiopathic seizures, patients with a younger age at onset carried a better prognosis for remission.
- Goodridge and Shorvon's (1983) community-based study followed 6,000 newly diagnosed patients in the United Kingdom for a mean of 8 years. Seventy-three percent were in remission (2 years seizure-free). Remission at 10 years was three times higher for patients who achieved 5-year remission than for those who did not.
- The Department of Veterans Affairs (VA) cooperative studies (Mattson et al., 1996) used monotherapy with phenytoin, carbamazepine, valproate, phenobarbital, or primidone in newly diagnosed adult patients with partial epilepsy. After initiation of treatment, approximately 50% of patients remained seizure-free for 12 months if they had only generalized tonic-clonic seizures. If complex partial seizures were present, only 23–32% of patients were seizure-free for 12 months.
- A Nova Scotia population-based study (Camfield et al., 1997) followed 417 pediatric epilepsy patients for an average of 8 years (excluding patients with progressive neurologic deficits or absence seizures) and showed that 61% of children receiving one antiepileptic drug (AED) in the first year of treatment ($n = 345$) were seizure-free at the end of follow-up. Seventeen percent had inadequate control with their first AED and received a second AED; of these, 42% had a complete remission. The presence of neurologic deficits and complex partial seizures predicted failure of control with the first AED.
- A British National General Practice Study of epilepsy (Cockerell et al., 1997) followed newly diagnosed patients with epilepsy ($n = 564$; 75% age ≥ 15) for a median of 7.2 years. Overall, 54% achieved a 5-year terminal remission. Remission was more likely in patients with idiopathic seizures. Children and patients with partial seizures achieved slightly lower remission rates. Standardized mortality rate (SMR) was 3.0. SMR was 1.6 for idiopathic cases versus 4.3 for remote symptomatic cases.

- Elwes and Reynolds (1991) suggested that patients who came under control relatively late and had numerous seizures before being controlled had a worse prognosis for eventual remission. This could be interpreted as uncontrolled seizures having an adverse effect on the prognosis (possible kindling-like effect), but it could also reflect the intrinsic intractability of epilepsy in these patients.

Prognosis for Psychosocial Outcome

- A population-based Finnish study (Silanpää et al., 1998) followed 245 children with epilepsy (28% idiopathic, 22% cryptogenic, 50% remote symptomatic) for approximately 30 years (90% available for follow-up). The best predictors of remission (≥5 years seizure-free) were idiopathic epilepsy and rapid initial response to treatment (≥75% seizure reduction), which occurred in 64% of surviving patients (47% off AEDs). Twenty percent of the patients were dead at follow-up, and 89% (39 of 44) of these were not seizure-free before death. Seventy-five percent (33 of 44) had remote symptomatic epilepsy. Ninety-nine of the epilepsy patients, who had no other neurologic handicaps, showed a significantly greater risk of completing only 6 years of school (relative risk 2.13), being unemployed (relative risk, 3.76), or being unmarried (relative risk, 3.5) versus matched controls.
- Specific epileptic syndromes are associated with a poor prognosis both for remission and for neurologic/psychosocial outcome, whereas others have good prognoses. Table 2.1 illustrates these contrasts.
- Sander (1993) categorized epilepsy according to long-term outcome as follows:
  - Mild epilepsy that does not require treatment and remits within a short period (approximately 30% of patients)
  - Epilepsy easily controlled on AEDs that eventually remit (approximately 30% of patients)
  - Chronic epilepsy that responds only partially to AEDs and has a continuing tendency to relapse (approximately 20% of patients)
  - Chronic, unremitting epilepsy with little response to treatment (approximately 20% of patients)

Morbidity and Mortality in Epilepsy

- The *standardized mortality rates* (mortality rate compared with the general population on an age-adjusted basis) in epilepsy are two to four times higher than normal and are highest in the first 10 years after diagnosis, especially in the first year after diagnosis.
- Causes of death in epileptic patients:
  - Directly related to a seizure or status epilepticus (10%)
  - Accidents during a seizure (5%)
  - Suicide (7–22%)
  - Sudden unexpected death in epilepsy (SUDEP) (>10%)

TABLE 2.1 Epilepsies with Good or Poor Prognosis for Seizure Remission and/or Neurologic Deterioration

Good Prognosis	*Poor Prognosis*
Childhood-onset absence seizures (idiopathic generalized "cortico-reticular" epilepsy)	*West syndrome
Benign epilepsies of childhood (including benign rolandic and benign occipital epilepsy, benign neonatal convulsions)	*Early infantile epileptic encephalopathies
Epilepsy in the elderly	*Neonatal convulsions
Febrile seizures	*Severe myoclonic epilepsy of infancy
Benign idiopathic neonatal convulsions	*Epilepsy partialis continua
	*Lennox-Gastaut
	*Landau-Kleffner syndrome (acquired epileptic aphasia)
	*Progressive myoclonus epilepsy (various types)
	Juvenile myoclonic epilepsy
	Temporal lobe epilepsy
	Nonconvulsive generalized status epilepticus
	Epilepsy due to cortical dysplasias

*Prognosis is poor for neurologic/mental deterioration.

- Characteristics of SUDEP:
  - Diagnosis of exclusion.
  - Incidence approximately 1–2 cases per 1,000 epileptic individuals per year.
  - Mean age 30–32 years.
  - Predominance in males.
  - One-third die in bed.
  - Alcohol abuse increases risk.
  - Seizure frequency *not* a risk factor.
  - Most have secondarily generalized tonic-clonic seizures.
  - Almost all have subtherapeutic antiepileptic blood levels.
  - Possible mechanisms: central autonomic overstimulation producing neurogenic pulmonary edema; cardiac arrhythmia; postseizure cessation of cerebral electrical activity.
- Accidents during seizures:
  - There is an increased risk of drowning (including bathtub drowning) and of burns (from cooktops, open flames, hot liquids, irons, curling irons, hot baths, showers, etc.).
  - Fractures include bilateral or unilateral posterior humeral fracture/dislocations, lumbar vertebral fractures, jaw fractures, facial fractures, and skull fractures.

- Accidents may occur during absence and complex partial seizures, as well as during atonic, myoclonic, and generalized tonic-clonic seizures (Wirrell et al., 1996).

Suggested Reading

Epidemiology and Prognosis of Epilepsy

Annegers JF. Epidemiology and genetics of epilepsy. Neurol Clin 1994;12:15-29.

Annegers JF, Hauser WA, Elveback LR. Remission of seizures and relapse in patients with epilepsy. Epilepsia 1979;20:729-739.

Berg AT, Testa FM, Levy SR, et al. The epidemiology of epilepsy: past, present and future. Neurol Clin 1996;14:383-398.

Camfield PR, Camfield CS, Gordon K, et al. If a first drug fails to control a child's epilepsy, what are the chances of success with the second drug? J Pediatr 1997;131:821-824.

Cockerell OC, Johnson AL, Sander JW, et al. Remission of epilepsy: results from the National General Practice Study of Epilepsy. Lancet 1995;346:140-144.

Cockerell OC, Johnson AL, Sander JW, et al. Prognosis of epilepsy: a review and further analysis of the first nine years of the British National General Practice Study of Epilepsy, a prospective population-based study. Epilepsia 1997;38:31-46.

Elwes RDC, Reynolds EH. The Early Prognosis of Epilepsy. In M Dam, L Gram (eds), Comprehensive Epileptology. New York: Raven, 1991;715-727.

Goodridge DMG, Shorvon SD. Epileptic seizures in a population of 6,000. II: treatment and prognosis. BMJ 1983;287:645-647.

Hauser WA. Seizure disorders: the changes with age. Epilepsia 1992;33(Suppl 4):S6-S14.

Hauser WAJ. Risk factors for epilepsy. Epilepsy Res 1991;4:45-52.

Hauser WAJ. Recent developments in the epidemiology of epilepsy. Acta Neurol Scand 1995;92(Suppl 162):17-21.

Hauser WA, Annegers JF, Rocca WA. Descriptive epidemiology of epilepsy: contributions of population-based studies from Rochester, Minnesota. Mayo Clin Proc 1996;71:576-586.

Hauser WA, Rich SS, Lee JRJ, et al. Risk of recurrent seizures after two unprovoked seizures. N Engl J Med 1998;38:429-434.

Mattson RH, Cramer JA, Collins JF, and the Department of Veterans Affairs Epilepsy Cooperative Studies No. 118 and No. 264 Group. Prognosis for total control of complex partial and secondarily generalized tonic-clonic seizures. Neurology 1996;47:68-76.

Sander JWAS. Some aspects of prognosis in the epilepsies: a review. Epilepsia 1993;34:1007-1016.

Silanpää M, Jalava M, Kaleva O, et al. Long-term prognosis of seizures with onset in childhood. N Engl J Med 1998;338:1715-1722.

Morbidity and Mortality in Epilepsy

Borchert LD, Labar DR. Permanent hemiparesis due to partial status epilepticus. Neurology 1995;45:187-188.

Cockerell OC. The mortality of epilepsy. Curr Opin Neurol 1996;9:93-96.

Cockerell OC, Johnson AL, Sander JW, et al. Mortality from epilepsy: results from a prospective population-based study. Lancet 1994;344:918-921.

Finelli PF, Cardi JK. Seizure as a cause of fracture. Neurology 1989;39:858-860.

Janz D. Neurological morbidity of severe epilepsy. Epilepsia 1988;29(Suppl 1):S1-S8.

Kirby S, Sadler MR. Injury and death as a result of seizures. Epilepsia 1995;36:25-28.

Lathers CM, Schraeder PL. Epilepsy and Sudden Death. New York: Marcel Dekker, 1990.

Leestma JE, Annegers JF, Brodie MJ, et al. Sudden unexplained death in epilepsy: observations from a large clinical development program. Epilepsia 1997;38:47-55.

Lesser RP, Lüders H, Wyllie E, et al. Mental deterioration in epilepsy. Epilepsia 1986;27 (Suppl 2):S105-S123.

Nashef L, Brown SW (eds). Epilepsy and sudden death. Epilepsia 1997;38(Suppl 11): S1-S76.

Nashef L, Fish DR, Sander JW, Shorvon SD. Incidence of sudden unexpected death in an adult outpatient cohort with epilepsy at a tertiary referral centre. J Neurol Neurosurg Psychiatry 1995;58:462-464.

Russell-Jones DL, Shorvon SD. The frequency and consequences of head injury in epileptic seizures. J Neurol Neurosurg Psychiatry 1989;52:659-662.

Terrence CF, Wisotzkey HM, Perper JA. Unexpected, unexplained death in epileptic patients. Neurology 1975;25:594-598.

Wirrell EC, Camfield PR, Camfield CS, et al. Accidental injury is a serious risk in children with typical absence epilepsy. Arch Neurol 1996;53:929-932.

3 Diagnosis

Diagnosis of epilepsy is a four-part process: (1) differentiation from events mimicking epileptic seizures, (2) seizure classification, (3) syndrome classification, and (4) determination of etiology (Figure 3.1).

Differential Diagnosis of Seizures

- Before appropriate AED therapy can be instituted, a diagnosis of epilepsy and a classification of seizure type(s) have to be made.
- A number of nonepileptic conditions, which must be distinguished from epileptic seizures, can present with alteration of consciousness, motor, sensory, or psychic symptoms (Tables 3.1–3.4).
- The two conditions most often mistaken for epileptic seizures are *syncope* and *nonepileptic psychogenic seizures* (pseudoseizures). Several features in the history of the patient or in the description of the attack may suggest nonepileptic seizures. Distinguishing features are outlined in Tables 3.5 and 3.6.
- In any epilepsy clinic, approximately 15% of intractable patients have pseudoseizures. Pseudoseizures occur concurrently with epilepsy in a minority of cases. Pseudoseizures may resemble any type of true epileptic seizure, though "convulsive" pseudoseizures are the most common. Pseudoseizure "status" is well described, and such patients are often admitted to intensive care units (Levitan and Bruni, 1986).
- Intensive EEG/video outpatient monitoring (see Chapter 4) is a useful technique for differentiating nonepileptic from epileptic seizures, provided the attacks occur frequently enough to provide opportunities to record them in the laboratory or provided they can reliably be provoked by specific stimuli or circumstances.
- Home videos of attacks taken by relatives can often be helpful.

Classification of Seizures and Epilepsy Syndromes

- Seizures and epilepsy syndromes are classified according to classifications of the International League Against Epilepsy (Tables 3.7 and 3.8).

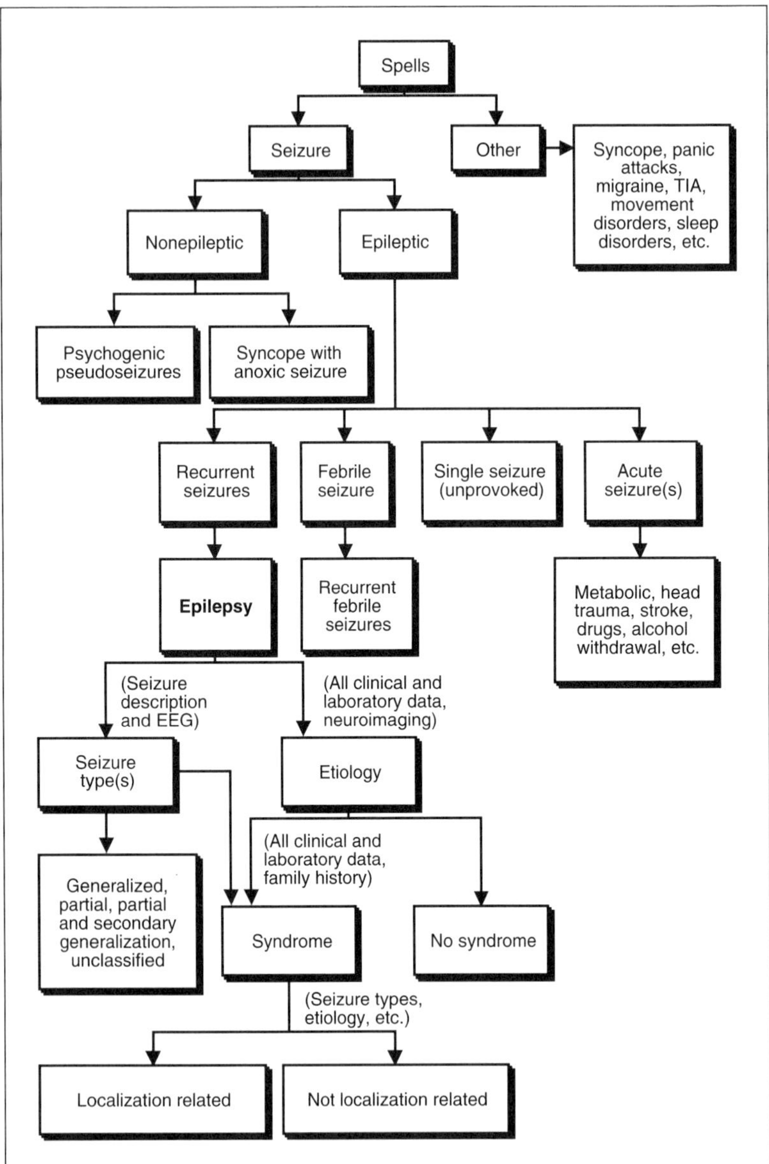

FIGURE 3.1 Algorithm for the diagnosis of seizures and epilepsy. (TIA = transient ischemic attack; EEG = electroencephalogram.)

TABLE 3.1 Conditions That May Result in Apparent Alteration or Loss of Consciousness

Syncope
Transient cerebral ischemia
Metabolic disorders (e.g., hypoglycemia)
Narcolepsy
Intermittent obstruction to cerebrospinal fluid flow (e.g., colloid cyst of third ventricle)
Drugs
Migraine
Psychiatric conditions
Pseudoseizures
Panic attacks
Dissociative or fugue states

- *Seizure classification* is based on *clinical features* of the ictal event and *EEG* features (ictal and interictal).
- Classification of *epilepsies and epilepsy syndromes* takes into consideration a number of clinical features that help better classify patients. These include type(s) of seizure(s), age of onset, neurologic development, precipitating factors, etiology, severity, chronicity, family history, diurnal pattern, response to drug therapy, EEG findings, and prognosis.
- In many cases, patients do not fit into a specific syndrome.
- Syndromes are more commonly identified, but more varied, in the pediatric epilepsy population.
- Specific epilepsy syndromes may respond best to particular AEDs.

Classification of Seizures

Partial Seizures

- Focal EEG features frequently
- Variety of clinical symptoms used to localize epileptic focus
- *Simple partial seizures*: generally brief and not associated with alteration of consciousness; may progress to complex partial or become secondarily generalized
- *Complex partial seizures*: associated with altered consciousness, in some cases, a complete lack of contact with the environment; may progress to secondarily generalized seizures

Generalized Seizures

- Generalized EEG features, bilaterally synchronous onset

TABLE 3.2 Conditions That May Present with Motor or Sensory Disturbances

Pseudoseizures
Transient ischemic attacks
Movement disorders (e.g., paroxysmal choreoathetosis/dystonia, paroxysmal kinesigenic choreoathetosis*)
Tics
Hyperexplexia
Nonepileptic myoclonus
Vestibular disturbances
Cataplexy
Tonic attacks of multiple sclerosis
Hemifacial spasm
Rapid eye movement (REM) and non-REM sleep disorders, parasomnias
Benign nocturnal myoclonus
Restless leg syndrome

*Paroxysmal kinesigenic choreoathetosis/dystonia:

- Controversial whether this is an epileptic or involuntary movement disorder.
- Onset usually in teens or 20s; may spontaneously remit or be life-long.
- Spells precipitated by sudden movement (e.g., getting up from a chair) or startle.
- Attacks last from seconds to minutes, rarely hours.
- Usually unilateral or asymmetric but can be bilateral.
- Mixed dystonia, choreoathetosis, or ballism.
- Idiopathic or secondary (e.g., stroke, encephalitis, hypocalcemia/hypo- or pseudo-hypoparathyroidism, multiple sclerosis).
- Familial or sporadic.
- Electroencephalography normal even during attack.
- Usually responds to small doses of carbamazepine.

- No focal features clinically (though myoclonic seizures may be asymmetric) and characterized by diffuse cerebral involvement
- Several clinical types (see Table 3.7)

Major Epilepsy Syndromes

Some of the well-defined or more common syndromes are discussed here (see Table 3.8). Other syndromes are mentioned under genetic etiology.

Generalized, Idiopathic (Genetic)

Childhood Absence Epilepsy

- Absence seizures, generally begin between ages 3 and 10 years.
- Genetic predisposition (multifactorial).

TABLE 3.3 Conditions That May Cause Drop Attacks

Seizures
- Atonic, tonic, myoclonic, myoclonic-atonic
- Partial seizures occasionally

Vascular insufficiency
- Anterior circulation ischemia
- Vertebrobasilar ischemia
- Spinal cord ischemia

Vestibular disorders
Cardiac arrhythmias (decreased cardiac output)
Movement-induced dystonias
Cataplexy
Hydrocephalus
Peripheral neuropathy
Parkinsonism
Postural instability in the elderly
Psychogenic
Unknown

- Patients are otherwise neurologically normal.
- More common in females.
- Multiple attacks tend to occur in the same day.
- Attacks generally are *typical* absences (Tables 3.9 and 3.10).
- Eyelid myoclonus common.
- Up to 50% develop tonic-clonic seizures, often around adolescence.
- Factors that increase likelihood of developing tonic-clonic seizures: (1) cognitive abnormality, (2) polyspike-wave on EEG, (3) later age of onset of absences, (4) photosensitivity, and (5) resistance of absences to treatment.
- EEG demonstrates generalized, bisynchronous symmetric 2- to 4-Hz spike and wave activity ictally and also in short interictal bursts; normal background.
- Often photo- and hyperventilation-sensitive.

TABLE 3.4 Conditions That Present with Psychic Symptoms

Hysteria
Episodic dyscontrol
Schizophreniform psychosis
Panic attacks
Drugs

TABLE 3.5 Syncope versus Epileptic Seizure

Characteristic	*Syncope*	*Epileptic Seizure*
Position	Usually upright (vasodepressor)	Any
Diurnal pattern	Daytime	Daytime or nighttime
Color	Pallor	Normal or cyanotic (tonic-clonic)
Aura	Dizziness, light-headedness, visual blurring or loss	Possible specific aura
Onset	Gradual (vasodepressor), occasionally sudden	Sudden or brief aura
Autonomic features	Common (vasodepressor)	Uncommon
Duration	Brief	Brief or prolonged
Injury	Rare	Can occur (tonic-clonic, atonic, myoclonic, tonic)
Urinary incontinence	Rare	More common
Disorientation, postictal	Rare	Can occur with tonic-clonic, complex partial
Motor activity	Occasionally brief tonic seizure or clonic jerks	Variable
Automatisms	None	Can occur with absence or complex partial
Electroenceph-alography	Normal interictally, slowing and flattening during the episode	Frequently abnormal ictally and interictally, may be normal

Note: A brief anoxic seizure may follow a syncopal episode. A temporal lobe seizure may rarely cause sinus arrest leading to a syncopal attack. Urinary incontinence is not a distinguishing feature.

- Generally good response to treatment (ethosuximide or valproate).
- Favorable prognosis by adulthood (seizures usually disappear by age 20).

Juvenile Absence Epilepsy

- Onset around puberty or early adolescence.
- No sex predominance.
- Genetic predisposition.
- Less frequent attacks than in childhood-onset absences.
- Up to 80% develop tonic-clonic seizures and often present with tonic-clonic seizures before absences.
- EEG demonstrates generalized spike and wave complexes.
- Good response to treatment.

TABLE 3.6 Epileptic Seizures versus Psychogenic Nonepileptic Seizures: Attack Characteristics

Characteristic	*Epileptic Seizure*	*Psychogenic Nonepileptic Seizure*
Age	Any	Any, less common in elderly
Aura	±	±
Triggers	Uncommon	Emotional disturbance
Duration	Brief	May be prolonged
Motor activity	Stereotypic, synchronous movements Automatisms in complex partial seizures Face involved	Rigidity Opisthotonus Avoidance behavior Irregular extremity movements, intermittent Forced eye closure Pelvic thrusting Side-to-side head movements Crying
Presence of others	Variable	Frequently
Diurnal pattern	Day or night	Usually day, never during sleep
Urinary incontinence	May occur	Rare
Physical injury	May occur	Rare
Reproduction of attack by suggestion	No	Suggestion alone or with such stimuli as tuning fork applied to forehead with suggestion
Electroencephalography	Interictal discharges frequent Ictal patterns almost always seen except for simple partial seizures or frontal lobe complex partial seizures; usually postictal slowing	Normal ictal and postictal patterns Epileptiform patterns may occur with concurrent epilepsy

Note: Complex partial seizures of frontal lobe origin may be difficult to distinguish from nonepileptic seizures.

TABLE 3.7 International Classification of Epileptic Seizures

I. Partial (focal, localized) seizures
  - Simple partial seizures
    - With motor signs
    - With somatosensory or special sensory systems
    - With autonomic symptoms or signs
    - With psychic symptoms
  - Complex partial seizures
    - Simple partial onset followed by impairment of consciousness
    - With impairment of consciousness at onset
  - Partial seizures evolving to secondarily generalized seizures
    - Simple partial seizures evolving to generalized seizures
    - Complex partial seizures evolving to generalized seizures
    - Simple partial seizures evolving to complex partial seizures evolving to generalized seizures

II. Generalized seizures (convulsive or nonconvulsive)
  - Absence seizures
    - Typical absences
    - Atypical absences
  - Myoclonic seizures
  - Clonic seizures
  - Tonic seizures
  - Tonic-clonic seizures
  - Atonic seizures (astatic seizures)

III. Unclassified epileptic seizures

Source: Commission on Classification and Terminology of the International League Against Epilepsy. Proposal for revised clinical and electroencephalographic classification of epileptic seizures. Epilepsia 1981;22:489–501.

- Prognosis favorable but probably less favorable than for childhood absence epilepsy.

Juvenile Myoclonic Epilepsy

- Probably the most common form of primary generalized epilepsy.
- Annual incidence 1–3 per 1,000 individuals.
- Family history of epilepsy in approximately 40%.
- Inheritance pattern can be autosomal recessive or dominant; gene likely localized on chromosome 6 in some families.
- Patients are otherwise neurologically normal.
- Onset of seizures typically between ages 8 and 18; peak incidence at age 15.
- Thirty percent of patients develop myoclonic, tonic-clonic, clonic-tonic-clonic, and absence seizures.
- Diagnosis at onset may be difficult if myoclonus has not developed.

TABLE 3.8 International Classification of Epilepsies, Epileptic Syndromes, and Related Seizure Disorders

- I. Localization-related (focal, local, partial)
  - Idiopathic (primary)
    - Benign childhood epilepsy with centrotemporal spikes
    - Childhood epilepsy with occipital paroxysms
    - Primary reading epilepsy
  - Symptomatic (secondary)
    - Temporal lobe epilepsies
    - Frontal lobe epilepsies
    - Parietal lobe epilepsies
    - Occipital lobe epilepsies
    - Chronic progressive epilepsia partialis continua of childhood
    - Syndromes characterized by seizures with specific modes of precipitation
  - Cryptogenic, defined by
    - Seizure type
    - Clinical features
    - Etiology
    - Anatomic localization
- II. Generalized
  - Idiopathic (primary)
    - Benign neonatal familial convulsions
    - Benign neonatal convulsions
    - Benign myoclonic epilepsy in infancy
    - Childhood absence epilepsy (pyknolepsy)
    - Juvenile absence epilepsy
    - Juvenile myoclonic epilepsy (impulsive petit mal)
    - Epilepsies with grand mal seizures on awakening
    - Other generalized idiopathic epilepsies
    - Epilepsies with seizures precipitated by specific modes of activation
  - Cryptogenic or symptomatic
    - West syndrome (infantile spasms, Blitz-Nick-Salaam Krämpfe)
    - Lennox-Gastaut syndrome
    - Epilepsy with myoclonic-astatic seizures
    - Epilepsy with myoclonic absences
  - Symptomatic (secondary)
    - Nonspecific cause
      - Early myoclonic encephalopathy
      - Early infantile epileptic encephalopathy with suppression bursts
      - Other symptomatic generalized epilepsies
    - Specific syndromes
      - Epileptic seizures may complicate many disease states
- III. Undetermined epilepsies
  - With both generalized and focal seizures
    - Neonatal seizures
    - Severe myoclonic epilepsy in infancy

TABLE 3.8 *Continued*

Epilepsy with continuous spike waves during slow-wave sleep
Acquired epileptic aphasia (Landau-Kleffner syndrome)
Other undetermined epilepsies
Without unequivocal generalized or focal features
IV. Special syndromes
Situation-related seizures (Gelegenheitsanfälle)
Febrile convulsions
Isolated seizures or isolated status epilepticus
Seizures occurring only with an acute or toxic event, due to factors such as alcohol, drugs, eclampsia, and nonketotic hyperglycemia

Source: Commission on Classification and Terminology of the International League Against Epilepsy. Proposal for a revised classification of epilepsies and epileptic syndromes. Epilepsia 1989;30:389-399.

- Sleep deprivation, stress, alcohol, and photosensitivity may be triggering or exacerbating factors.
- Myoclonic and generalized tonic-clonic seizures tend to occur in early morning, after a nap, or nocturnally.
- EEG demonstrates generalized spike-wave and polyspike-wave activity typically at 4-6 Hz with normal background; focal abnormalities or asymmetries may be seen in 50% of patients.
- Excellent response to therapy (80% controlled on valproate).
- In patients failing valproate, carbamazepine may control the generalized tonic-clonic seizures, but it can exacerbate the myoclonus.
- Lamotrigine or topiramate are possible alternatives.
- Prognosis for remission of seizures is poor: When AED therapy is discontinued, relapse rate is 90%.

Generalized, Symptomatic

West Syndrome (Infantile Spasms)

- Epilepsy syndrome with seizures starting in the first year of life (usually 3-5 months of age).
- Incidence 2-4 per 100,000 live births.
- Spasms, most frequently flexor.
- Spasms may involve head, neck, and trunk and are usually generalized.
- Often associated with retarded mental development.
- A number of causes, including degenerative and metabolic disorders, cortical dysgenesis, neurocutaneous syndromes (especially tuberous sclerosis), or acquired lesions such as anoxia, infections, tumors, trauma, or hemorrhage; cryptogenic in 40-50%.

TABLE 3.9 Typical Absence versus Atypical Absence

Characteristic	*Typical*	*Atypical*
Duration	10–20 secs	Longer
Loss of consciousness	Complete	Often incomplete
Onset	Abrupt	Less abrupt
Termination	Abrupt	Less abrupt
Number of attacks	Multiple in a single day	Less frequent
Hyperventilation	Frequent trigger	Less frequent trigger
Photosensitivity	Can be present	Less frequent
Associated phenomena	Brief eyelid fluttering common	Automatisms more prominent Changes in muscle tone prominent Autonomic phenomena
Age	4–20 yrs	Any
Clinical setting	Idiopathic	Occur in symptomatic epilepsies Neurologic abnormalities Multiple seizure types
Electroencephalography	Normal background Bilateral, symmetric bisynchronous 2- to 4-Hz spike-wave activity	Abnormal background Asymmetric 2.0- to 2.5-Hz irregular spike wave Spike-sharp wave bursts Paroxysmal fast activity
Response to therapy	Favorable	Less favorable

- EEG: hypsarrhythmia, a disorganized pattern, bilateral asynchrony with high-voltage slow waves, and multifocal epileptic discharges predominating in posterior head regions; voltage depression during seizures.
- Spasms usually remit with treatment (e.g., vigabatrin, adrenocorticotropic hormone).
- Long-term prognosis poor; frequent mental retardation, continuing epilepsy; may evolve into Lennox-Gastaut syndrome.
- Some cases, often with asymmetric seizures, have shown focal brain abnormalities on positron emission tomography (PET) or magnetic resonance imaging (MRI), and clinical improvement with surgical removal of the focus (e.g., cortical tubers).

Lennox-Gastaut Syndrome

- Usual onset in childhood (1–8 years of age); rare onset in adolescence.
- Multiple causes, including developmental abnormalities, encephalitis, tuberous sclerosis, metabolic disorders, birth hypoxia, or vascular injury; 25% cryptogenic.

TABLE 3.10 Absence versus Complex Partial Seizures

Characteristic	*Absence*	*Complex Partial*
Neurologic status	Normal	May have positive history or examination
Age	Usually childhood	Any age
Duration	Seconds	Minutes; frontal lobe origin, seconds
Onset	Abrupt	May have a brief aura
Termination	Abrupt	May have brief period of disorientation postictally
Frequency	Frequent	Less frequent
Automatisms	May occur if duration >10 secs	Common
	Less complex	More complex automatisms may be observed
Provocation by hyperventilation	Common	Uncommon
Electroencephalography	Generalized 2- to 4-Hz spike-wave	May be normal, focal spikes/sharp waves interictally
Etiology	Idiopathic/genetic (most commonly)	Cryptogenic, symptomatic (multiple etiologies)
Neuroimaging studies	Normal	May be abnormal (e.g., mesial temporal abnormalities)
Response to anti-epilepsy drugs	Usually good	Often resistant

- May evolve from West syndrome or an ongoing epileptic encephalopathy.
- Secondarily generalized form of epilepsy.
- Mental impairment.
- Multiple seizure types.
- Seizures may be atonic, axial tonic (including tonic status during sleep), myoclonic, atypical absence, or tonic-clonic.
- Drop attacks may occur with tonic, atonic, or myoclonic seizures and often lead to injury.
- Seizures difficult to control.
- Status epilepticus common, especially atypical absence status.
- EEG: abnormal background and abundant slow spike and wave activity (1.0–2.5 Hz); 10-Hz rapid rhythms during sleep.
- Prognosis poor.
- Most commonly used AEDs: valproate, phenytoin, lamotrigine, clobazam, clonazepam, topiramate; also ketogenic diet.

Benign Neonatal Convulsions

- This syndrome is not clearly partial or generalized.
- Some cases are familial, autosomal dominant; locus on long arm of chromosome 20, but with some heterogeneity.
- In cases with family history, seizures usually occur on the second or third days of life.
- In cases with no family history, seizures usually occur around the fifth day of life.
- Seizures are usually brief.
- Infants are neurologically normal.
- Generally good prognosis. Late epilepsy may occur in 15% of patients with familial variety.
- EEG in familial variety shows no specific pattern.
- In nonfamilial variety, EEG abnormality consists of bursts of theta that are often asynchronous.

Progressive Myoclonus Epilepsies

- This is a group of disorders with various etiologies having the common feature of myoclonus and epilepsy.
- Usually progressive neurologic deterioration.
- Most are due to inherited metabolic abnormalities.
- Causes and features are shown in Table 3.11.

Localization-Related

The following *benign* partial epilepsy syndromes of childhood are not associated with focal brain lesions, have normal neuroimaging studies, and generally have good prognoses. They must be distinguished from other partial epilepsies secondary to structural pathology.

Benign Rolandic Epilepsy (Benign Partial Epilepsy with Centrotemporal Spikes)

- A childhood epilepsy syndrome with seizures generally occurring between 3 and 15 years of age.
- Annual incidence is 10–11 per 100,000 individuals younger than age 15.
- Seizures ("sylvian seizures") are usually partial, involving face, oropharyngeal structures, and arm. Speech arrest, facial twitching, oral-buccal-lingual paresthesias, choking, vomiting, or a combination thereof is seen.
- Secondarily generalized tonic-clonic seizures are rare.
- Seizures tend to occur nocturnally.
- Epilepsy is generally mild and may not require treatment; seizures are usually infrequent.
- Normal intelligence and neurologic status.
- Genetic factors important in etiology.
- EEG demonstrates unilateral or bilateral focal centrotemporal spikes, with a horizontal dipole that is accentuated during sleep.

TABLE 3.11 Most Common Causes of Progressive Myoclonus Epilepsy

Syndrome	*Age of Onset*	*Genetics/Pathology*	*Clinical Features/Prognosis*
MERRF (myoclonus epilepsy and ragged red fibers)	Variable	Point mutation in tRNA gene of maternally derived mitochondrial genome, familial or sporadic	Intention myoclonus, epilepsy, deafness, optic atrophy, myopathy, lipomas, dementia, neuropathy, wide clinical spectrum
Baltic myoclonus (Unverricht-Lundborg)	6–15 yrs	Autosomal recessive locus at 21q22-3; gene coding for the protein cystatin-B; neuronal loss and gliosis of cerebellum, medial thalamus, spinal cord; high incidence in Baltic region, also Southern Europe, North Africa	Onset with stimulus-sensitive myoclonus and generalized tonic-clonic seizures, mild dementia, ataxia, variable rate of progression
Lafora body disease	11–18 yrs	Autosomal recessive locus at 6q23–25; polyglucosan inclusions in neurons, heart and skeletal muscle, liver, eccrine sweat gland duct cells	Asymmetric myoclonus, generalized tonic-clonic seizures, focal occipital seizures, progressive dementia, apraxia, visual loss, usual death within 5 yrs of onset
Dentato-pallidoluysian atrophy	Childhood or adolescence	Autosomal dominant; chromosome 12p; CAG triplet repeat; mainly in Japan	Chorea, ataxia, dementia, myoclonus, seizures
Lipidoses (lysosomal storage diseases)	—	—	—
Tay-Sachs (GM_2-gangliosidosis)	3–6 mos	Autosomal recessive, mainly Ashkenazi Jews, mutation at 15q23–24, hexosaminidase A deficiency	Stimulus-sensitive myoclonus, blindness, cherry red spot, hypotonia, developmental regression, later: megalencephaly, spasticity, death by ~4 yrs

Sandhoff's (0 variant of Tay-Sachs)	3–6 mos	Lack of both hexosaminidase A and B, chromosome 5	Similar clinical picture to Tay-Sachs plus hepatosplenomegaly
Gaucher's type 3	Preadolescence	Autosomal recessive, β-glucocerebrosidase deficiency, chromosome 1q21–22	Hepatosplenomegaly, dementia, spasticity, myoclonus, foam cells in bone marrow
Sialidosis type I (cherry red spot–myoclonus syndrome)	Adolescence; late childhood	Autosomal recessive, deficient glycoprotein acid α-neuraminidase	Cherry red spot in fundus, stimulus-sensitive myoclonus, ataxia, vision loss
Neuronal ceroid lipofuscinosis	—	Inclusion bodies on EM in neurons and eccrine sweat glands: curvilinear fingerprint body, granular osmophilic deposits	—
Infantile/late infantile (Haltia-Santavuori, Jansky-Bielschowsky, Finnish variant)	2–4 yrs	Autosomal recessive; Finnish variety linked to chromosome 1p	Various seizure types, psychomotor regression, ataxia, visual loss; death in ~5 yrs
Juvenile (Batten, Spielmeyer-Vogt-Sjögren)	4–10 yrs	Autosomal recessive; chromosome 16p12	Seizures (not prominent), vision loss, dementia, extrapyramidal; variable course; death in ~8 yrs
Adult (Kufs')	~30 yrs	Autosomal recessive	Dementia; usually death in ~12 yrs

EM = electron microscopy.

- Excellent response to treatment.
- Excellent prognosis (usually disappears by age 15).

Benign Occipital Epilepsy

- Age of onset is 1–14 years (most between ages 4 and 8).
- May occur with or evolve into benign rolandic epilepsy.
- Neurologically normal children.
- Migraine-like headaches and vomiting are common, especially in younger patients.
- Visual phenomena occur: loss of vision, scintillations, phosphenes, formed visual hallucinations, and illusions.
- Seizures may be adversive, oculoclonic, hemiclonic, generalized tonic-clonic, or complex partial.
- EEG: unilateral or bilateral posterior spike-wave activated by sleep; may be suppressed by eye closure; may be photosensitive.
- Prognosis: usually remits by teens; earlier onset patients have a better prognosis.

Other Benign Partial Epilepsy Syndromes of Childhood

- Benign partial epilepsy with frontal spikes
- Benign epilepsy with extreme somatosensory evoked potentials
- Benign complex partial epilepsy

Frontal Lobe Epilepsy

- Simple or complex partial with or without secondary generalization.
- Complex partial seizures of frontal lobe origin are briefer, more abrupt in onset and termination, and occur with greater frequency than complex partial seizures of temporal lobe origin.
- Auras are often nonspecific.
- Vocalizations or speech arrest can occur.
- Bizarre bimanual/bipedal activity, often from onset.
- Automatisms may be bizarre and may be mistaken for nonepileptic seizures.
- Sexual automatisms can be seen.
- May be associated with falls.
- Adversive head or eye deviation may occur.
- Frontal complex partial seizures have a tendency to be nocturnal.
- May occur in clusters.
- Complex partial status is relatively common.
- Secondary generalization is more common than with temporal complex partial seizures.
- Postictal Todd's paralysis frequent, with onset near motor cortex.
- EEG frequently normal, even ictally.
- Neuroimaging studies often negative, localization often difficult.
- Responds less well to surgery than temporal seizures.
- *Supplementary motor seizures* consist of speech arrest and movement of eyes and head toward the extended, abducted arm.

- *Jacksonian motor seizures* (after Hughlings Jackson) consist of a march of clonic activity from one body part to another, corresponding to the spread of discharge along the precentral motor strip.

Temporal Lobe/Temporolimbic Epilepsy

- Onset in early childhood.
- Seizures typically disappear for several years and return in teens or early adulthood.
- History of febrile convulsions, especially complex febrile seizures. History of febrile convulsions found in approximately 40% of cases of intractable temporal lobe epilepsy.
- Features of mesial temporal sclerosis apparent on neuroimaging.
- Simple or complex partial, with or without secondary generalization.
- Auras are very common—for example, epigastric sensations, autonomic features, psychic symptoms such as fear (amygdalar involvement), déjà vu, jamais vu, olfactory/gustatory (uncus involvement), visual phenomena.
- Frequently associated with automatisms: oroalimentary, vocalizations, repetitive movements, and complex activities.
- Dystonic posturing of one limb may occur contralateral to the focus.
- Neocortical temporal lobe epilepsy may show aphasic features, vomiting (right temporal), auditory symptoms, visual phenomena, and more prominent motor activity than with mesial-basal seizures. However, rapid spread often produces features similar to temporolimbic seizures.
- Secondary generalization less common than with frontal lobe seizures.
- Seizure frequency less than with frontal lobe-onset complex partial seizures.
- Complex partial status less frequent than in frontal seizures.
- Resistant to AEDs.
- When mesial temporal sclerosis identified, excellent response to temporal lobectomy (in greater than 80% of cases).

Parietal Lobe Epilepsy

- Simple partial, motor, or sensory, with or without secondary generalization.
- Usually positive phenomena (e.g., paresthesias, tingling).
- Frequently involve face, arm, or hand.
- Jacksonian somatosensory seizures involve a march of symptoms corresponding to a spread of the discharge along the sensory homunculus in the postcentral gyrus.
- Rotatory movements can occur.
- Painful epileptic seizures, which are rare.
- Visual phenomena may consist of formed hallucinations.
- Dominant hemisphere involvement may result in language disturbances.

Occipital Lobe Epilepsy

- Usually simple partial with visual symptoms, with or without secondary generalization.

- Visual symptoms are elementary (e.g., flashes of light, color, and patterns) unlike the more complex visual hallucinations of posterior parietal or posterior temporal lobe origin.
- Ictal blindness.
- Contralateral conjugate eye deviation with nystagmus.

Rasmussen's Encephalitis

Rasmussen's encephalitis is a rare syndrome that is quite distinct and important to recognize because of its potential treatability.

- Usually begins between 14 months and 14 years of age; very rare adult-onset cases.
- Onset of drug-resistant partial seizures with progressive unilateral motor deficit; epilepsia partialis continua may occur.
- Progressive cerebral hemiatrophy seen on MRI.
- Intellectual deterioration.
- Variable course.
- EEG demonstrates polymorphic delta activity, loss of normal background rhythms, and frequent spike discharges that have unilateral predominance and may be periodic.
- Pathology shows glial nodules with perivascular lymphocytic cuffing.
- Surgical resection (functional hemispherectomy) may be helpful if disease becomes stabilized.
- Antibodies to GluR3 (a glutamate receptor subunit) have been identified in some patients, suggesting an autoimmune pathogenesis.
- Evidence of cytomegalovirus infection has been found in some patients' brains, and response to ganciclovir has been reported.
- IVIG and immune adsorption techniques have been tried with variable success.

Epilepsy with Bilateral Occipital Calcifications and Celiac Disease

- Found mainly in Italian patients but has been seen in patients of other origins.
- Epilepsy begins in childhood and usually consists of intractable, complex partial and secondarily generalized tonic-clonic seizures; some patients have evidence of occipital seizures with phenomena such as elementary visual hallucinations.
- Patients have symptomatic or asymptomatic celiac disease.
- Bilateral, usually crescentic symmetric calcifications are seen on computed tomographic (CT) scan. Occasionally, calcifications are more widespread (see Figure 4.19).
- Pathology reveals venous hemangiomas in deeper cortical layers, with subcortical calcification of vessel walls and gliosis.
- These patients do not have features of Sturge-Weber syndrome.

Reflex Epilepsies

- Seizures provoked by a specific mental or external stimulus (Table 3.12).
- May be partial, generalized tonic-clonic, or myoclonic.

- Syndromes classified as localization-related symptomatic seizures with specific modes of precipitation (e.g., musicogenic epilepsy, which may have a focus near Heschl's gyrus) or generalized seizures precipitated by specific modes of activation (e.g., primary reading epilepsy).
- Patients may also experience spontaneous seizures.
- Photosensitive seizures most common.
- Recommendations for patients with television (TV)-induced or photosensitive epilepsy: Stay at least 2 m from TV screen or 30 cm from computer monitor; do not adjust a flickering TV screen; watch TV in a well-lit room; consider covering one eye when watching TV or using a computer; avoid fluorescent and

TABLE 3.12 Triggering Factors in Reflex Epilepsies

Visual
Photic stimulation
Patterns
Television
Video games
Eye closure
Eye fluttering
Color
Auditory
Music (piece, note)
Specific voice
Specific sound
Somatosensory
Tap or touch
Hot water immersion
Tooth brushing
Mental (thinking)
Calculation
Problem solving (e.g., chess, math problems)
Card games
Drawing
Motor
Movement (kinesigenic)
Swallowing
Eye movements (convergence)
Other (combination)
Reading
Eating
Exercise
Being startled

strobe lights; avoid sunlight shimmering off water or flickering through trees; and wear sunglasses in bright light.

- Reading epilepsy may be primary generalized (generalized tonic-clonic seizures preceded by jaw myoclonus) or secondary due to a temporal focus. Some cases also have seizures provoked by other language tasks, such as reading aloud.
- Desensitizing techniques have been used successfully with some reflex epilepsies.

Undetermined and Situation-Related

Febrile Seizures

- Definition: generalized seizures occurring in association with fever and absence of central nervous system (CNS) infections. Seizures with fever in children with previous afebrile seizures are excluded.
- Occur in 3–4% of children between 3 months and 6 years of age, 90% prior to age 3. Peak incidence at 15 months for first febrile seizure.
- Genetic factors play a role. A genetic, generalized epilepsy syndrome with febrile seizures continuing after the conventional limit of 6 years of age and with additional nonfebrile absences, myoclonic, and generalized tonic-clonic seizures in neurologically normal individuals has been described. Febrile seizures are seen in 8% of siblings if one sibling has febrile seizures, and in 22% if a sibling and a parent had febrile seizures. Monozygotic twins have an approximately 40% concordance rate versus a 7% concordance rate for dizygotic twins. The mode of inheritance has been suggested as polygenic or multifactorial.
- Increased incidence in individuals with neurologic handicap from birth, family history of seizures, or febrile convulsions.
- Meningitis, if a consideration at time of presentation, must be ruled out by lumbar puncture. Lumbar puncture should be strongly considered in all children younger than 12 months.
- EEG is not indicated and is not a useful predictor of seizure recurrence or the development of epilepsy
- CT scan is not required in simple febrile seizures.
- Febrile seizures recur in 30–40% of cases.
- Ten percent experience three or more febrile seizures.
- Independent risk factors predicting likelihood of recurrence are
    - Young age at time of first febrile seizure (<15 months)
    - History of febrile seizures in a first-degree relative
    - Low degree of fever while in the emergency department
    - Brief duration between onset of fever and the first seizure

In 1997, Berg et al. reported a 70% risk of at least one recurrence with all of the above four risk factors present, versus a less than 20% chance of recurrence if none of the above risk factors was present.

- Attendance at day care also increases the likelihood of recurrence.
- Overall risk of subsequent epilepsy is 2–3%.
- Children who have a single, brief generalized seizure (simple febrile seizures), a negative family history of epilepsy, and no preexisting neurologic handicap have no or minimal increased risk of developing epilepsy. Recurrence of febrile seizures does not significantly increase the risk for subsequent epilepsy.
- With two or more of the following risk factors, there is a 6–15% chance of developing epilepsy.
  - Seizure duration greater than 15 minutes
  - Focal seizure
  - Abnormal preexisting neurologic status
  - Seizure recurrence in the first 24 hours
  - History of epilepsy in a parent or sibling
- Chronic AED treatment is generally not recommended, nor is overuse of over-concern about antipyretic treatment.
- Parental reassurance and education are important parts of management.
- When seizures occur, rectal diazepam (0.5 mg/kg) can be given by a 3-ml syringe using the IV diazepam formulation (or diazepam rectal gel). Respirations should be monitored for 30 minutes.
- Diazepam administration is most useful for children who habitually have prolonged febrile seizures or who live far from health care facilities.
- A 1998 report from Verity et al. showed that 10-year-old children who have simple or complex febrile seizures but who are neurologically normal otherwise perform as well as controls on tests of intellect or behavior.

Severe Myoclonic Epilepsy of Infancy

- Onset before 12 months of age, usually with fever.
- Generalized or unilateral clonic seizures (may alternate sides).
- Myoclonic jerks begin between 12 and 36 months of age.
- Initially neurologically normal, followed by progressive cognitive decline and ataxia from the second year of life.
- To be differentiated from early infantile encephalopathies (Ohtahara syndrome and related disorders) that are often associated with cerebral malformations, perinatal hypoxia/ischemia or metabolic abnormalities (e.g., nonketotic hyperglycinemia), Ohtahara syndrome cases, as opposed to severe myoclonic epilepsy of infancy, have earlier onset, tonic extensor spasms, severely abnormal EEG with suppression bursts or hypsarrhythmia, and very poor prognosis.
- Etiology unknown, family history of epilepsy or febrile seizures common.
- EEG shows generalized spike-wave, polyspike-wave, and photosensitivity.
- Seizures resistant to treatment; poor prognosis.

Landau-Kleffner Syndrome

- Acquired aphasia with epilepsy in childhood.
- Onset at time of language acquisition.
- Failure of speech development.

- Psychomotor or behavioral disturbances.
- Male predominance.
- Epileptic seizures in 70%.
- EEG demonstrates paroxysmal activity over temporal or parieto-occipital regions that is activated during sleep.
- Etiology unknown.
- No neuroimaging abnormalities.
- AEDs and corticosteroids have partial effect on seizure control, but no significant effect on language function.

Etiologies of Epilepsy and Seizures

- Virtually any type of cerebral lesion affecting the cortex can cause epilepsy or seizures, including metabolic or molecular (e.g., ion channel or neurotransmitter receptor) abnormalities, which are often genetic (Tables 3.13 and 3.14).
- Gray matter structural lesions are much more likely to cause seizures/epilepsy than are pure white matter lesions. Whether seizures can arise from subcortical gray matter, such as the basal ganglia or thalamus, is not well established.
- Etiology is often multiple—a combination of acquired and genetic factors.
- Etiology is very much age-related.
  - *Newborn*: infectious, metabolic (e.g., pyridoxine dependency, hypoglycemia, hypocalcemia), birth anoxia or intracranial hemorrhage, major brain malformations
  - *Infants/young children*: febrile convulsions, inherited metabolic or developmental diseases, idiopathic/genetic syndromes, infectious, dysplasias, degenerative

TABLE 3.13 Etiology of Newly Diagnosed Epilepsy in Adults and Children (Excluding Neonates) from a Population-Based Study in the United Kingdom (*n* = 564)

Etiology	*Percent*
Unknown	62
Cerebrovascular	15
Alcohol-related	6
Cerebral tumor	6
Cerebral infection	2
Cerebral trauma	2
Other	6

Source: JWAS Sander, YM Hart, AL Johnson, et al. The National General Practice Study of Epilepsy: newly diagnosed seizures in a general population. Lancet 1990;336:1267–1271.

TABLE 3.14 Presumed Etiology of Newly Diagnosed Epilepsy in Rochester, Minnesota, 1935–1984 (All Ages)

Etiology	*Percent*
Cryptogenic	68.7%
Known cause	31.3%
Cerebrovascular disease	13.2%
Developmental	5.5%
Brain trauma	4.1%
Brain tumor	3.6%
Cerebral infection	2.6%
Degenerative disease	1.8%
Other	0.5%

Source: Adapted from JF Annegers. Epidemiology and genetics of epilepsy. Neurol Clin 1994;12:15-29.

- *Older children/adolescents*: mesial temporal sclerosis, idiopathic/genetic syndromes, degenerative, dysplasias, trauma, tumors
- *Adults*: trauma, tumors, cerebrovascular, inherited metabolic, alcohol/drugs, mesial temporal sclerosis, infectious, multiple sclerosis, degenerative
- *Elderly*: cerebrovascular, drugs/alcohol, tumors, trauma, degenerative (e.g., Alzheimer's disease)

Genetic Factors

- The importance of genetic factors in epilepsy is shown by the 95% concordance rate in monozygotic twins versus the 15% concordance rate in dizygotic twins.
- Overall risk of unprovoked seizures in offspring of a parent with epilepsy is approximately 6% (twice as high in maternal than paternal epilepsy); risk rises to 9-12% in parents with idiopathic epilepsy.
- At least 141 single-gene disorders that cause brain abnormalities have epilepsy among their manifestations.
- Although genetic factors are most important in the idiopathic generalized epilepsies, they also figure to a degree in certain epilepsies or seizure syndromes with a strong environmental or "acquired" component, such as post-traumatic epilepsy and febrile convulsions.
- The following *chromosomal abnormalities* have epilepsy, or an increased risk of epilepsy, as one of their manifestations:
  - Trisomy 21 (Down syndrome, 2-15% prevalence of epilepsy). Various pathologies have been associated, including Alzheimer's changes in older patients.
  - Trisomy 13, 18, or 22 (epilepsy in 20-25%).

- Deletion of part of chromosome 4 (Wolf-Hirschhorn syndrome); seizures in 70%.
- Partial monosomy 5p (cri du chat).
- Ring chromosome 14.
- Ring chromosome 20.
- Extrastructural abnormal chromosome 15 syndrome.
- Deletion on the proximal portion on the long arm of maternally derived chromosome 15 (Angelman "happy puppet" syndrome).

- *Mitochondrial DNA disorders* (maternal inheritance) may have epilepsy and myoclonus (e.g., MERRF [myoclonic epilepsy and ragged red fibers] and MELAS [mitochondrial myopathy, encephalopathy, lactic acidosis, stroke-like episodes]). The epilepsy can be severe and intractable, with repeated bouts of status epilepticus.
- Some specified *inherited metabolic disorders* with an increased incidence of seizures:
  - Aminoacidopathies (e.g., phenylketonuria, nonketotic hyperglycinemia, maple syrup urine disease)
  - Galactosemia
  - Lysosomal lipid storage diseases (e.g., Tay-Sachs disease)
  - Leukodystrophies
  - Mucopolysaccharidoses (e.g., Sanfilippo's syndrome)
  - Peroxisomal disorders
  - Acute intermittent porphyria
  - Pyridoxine deficiency
  - Pseudohypoparathyroidism (Guberman and Jaworski, 1979)/hypoparathyroidism (may be acquired)
  - Wilson's disease (seizures unusual)
- Hereditary neurocutaneous disorders:
  - *Tuberous sclerosis*: Classic triad of adenoma sebaceum (facial angiofibromas), mental retardation (not in all cases), and epilepsy (in >80%). Infantile spasms, partial motor, complex partial, and secondarily generalized seizures are seen. Other features are periungual fibromata, cortical tubers, subependymal hamartomas (see Figure 4.18A), astrocytomas causing ventricular obstruction and hydrocephalus, renal angiomyolipomas, depigmented ash-leaf macules (see Figure 4.18B), and cardiac rhabdomyomas. It is autosomal dominant and linked to chromosome 9 or 16 in some families. The abnormal gene on chromosome 16 encodes a possible tumor suppressor protein called *tuberin*.
  - *Neurofibromatosis*: Epilepsy is uncommon (approximately 3–13%) in neurofibromatosis 1 (NF-1). It is autosomal dominant and localized to chromosome 17q. Epilepsy may be due to cerebral hamartoma, neuronal migration abnormalities, or gliomas, all of which can occur with NF-1. Generalized tonic-clonic, complex partial seizures or infantile spasms can occur.

  - *Sturge-Weber syndrome*: It is a nonhereditary, neurocutaneous disorder (port wine stain—usually of upper face, leptomeningeal venous angioma, buphthalmos) that causes seizures in 71–89% of cases. Seizures are usually partial motor with secondary generalization, begin in the first 2 years of life, are often intractable, and may require hemispherectomy.
- Seizures occur in 5–10% of adult-onset *Huntington's disease* patients. The genetic abnormality is an unstable CAG triplet expansion on chromosome 4p. Juvenile-onset patients have a higher incidence of seizures.
- Epilepsy due to stroke is usually relatively easy to control with AEDs.
- *Fragile X syndrome*: mental retardation, facial dysmorphism, and epilepsy in 20–40%; may resemble benign rolandic epilepsy. Unstable CGG triplet repeat at Xq28.
- Epilepsy occurs in 70–80% of cases of *Rett syndrome*, which affects girls, usually begins between ages 1 and 2 years. Features include developmental delay, loss of expressive language and purposeful hand movements, hand-wringing posture, autism, microcephaly, gait apraxia, and often a variety of seizure types, including reflex cortical myoclonus.
- Seizures are common in *Alpers' syndrome*, which may be autosomal recessive or sporadic, and which begins in infancy or childhood with developmental delay, failure to thrive, and liver failure. EEG shows high-amplitude, polyspike-slow waves.
- Specific epilepsy syndromes with heredofamilial basis but without clearly defined metabolic or structural abnormalities:
  - *Idiopathic generalized ("cortico-reticular") epilepsy* with childhood-onset absence seizures and, in some cases, generalized tonic-clonic seizures.
    - Concordance rate reaches 80% in monozygotic twins.
    - Phenotypic and EEG expression (3-Hz spike-wave) is age-specific, both usually disappearing by age 20.
    - Significantly increased incidence of epilepsy or EEG trait in first-degree relatives.
    - Risk of a child inheriting this form of epilepsy if one first-degree relative is affected is 5–20%.
    - Polygenic inheritance or autosomal dominant with variable penetrance is most likely.
  - *Benign rolandic epilepsy* (see Major Epilepsy Syndromes) of childhood is often familial.
- Epilepsy syndromes in which gene abnormalities have been described:
  - *Juvenile myoclonic epilepsy*: Unclear whether autosomal dominant or recessive pattern. Localization to short arm of chromosome 6 in some families.
  - *Benign familial neonatal convulsions* (see Major Epilepsy Syndromes): Rare autosomal dominant disorder. Convulsions begin on second or third day of life and resolve by 6 months of age. Some families linked to marker on long arm of chromosome 20 and others linked to chromosome 8. The abnormal gene is related to a voltage-gated potassium channel (Charlier et al., 1998).

- *Autosomal dominant nocturnal frontal lobe epilepsy* with a tendency toward seizures in sleep has been described and linked to chromosome 20. A missense point mutation in a gene coding the α subunit of the nicotinic acetylcholine receptor has been described.
- *Partial epilepsy with auditory symptoms*: Onset of auditory seizures (hum or ringing), complex partial seizures, or secondarily generalized tonic-clonic seizures between ages 8 and 19 years. Localized to chromosome 10q in at least one family.
- *Baltic myoclonus epilepsy* (progressive myoclonus epilepsy of Unverricht-Lundborg): Autosomal recessive, onset of stimulus-sensitive myoclonus and generalized tonic-clonic seizures between ages 6 and 15 years, mild dementia, ataxia, variable rate of progression. Tentatively localized to chromosome 21q. A mutation in the gene coding the protein cystatin B (a cysteine protease inhibitor) has been identified.

- *Progressive myoclonus epilepsy with Lafora bodies*: Autosomal recessive, onset in adolescence, myoclonus, progressive dementia, and neurologic deterioration leading to death. Has been linked to chromosome 6q.

Developmental Abnormalities

- Epilepsy occurs frequently with major prenatal or perinatal insults, leading to cerebral palsy. Mental retardation and motor deficits are frequent accompaniments.
- MRI and other neuroimaging techniques have allowed increasing recognition of cortical dysplasias (Table 3.15), some of which are quite subtle.
- Neuronal migration disorders commonly associated with epilepsy:
  - Congenital bilateral perisylvian polymicrogyria (developmental Foix-Chavany-Marie syndrome [see Figure 4.27])
  - Focal cortical dysplasia (of Taylor)
  - Lissencephaly (agyria-pachygyria)
  - X-linked lissencephaly and subcortical band heterotopia
  - X-linked bilateral periventricular nodular heterotopia (see Figure 4.28)
  - Band heterotopia (double cortex syndrome)—chromosome Xq22/3, mostly in females
  - Other neuronal heterotopias—chromosome Xq28
  - Hemimegalencephaly (see Figure 4.26)
  - Polymicrogyria
  - Sublobar dysplasia
  - Agenesis of the corpus callosum (see Figure 4.29)
- *Aicardi syndrome*: Agenesis of the corpus callosum, unlayered microgyria, periventricular and subcortical heterotopias, severe mental retardation, infantile spasms, chorioretinal lacunae occurring in girls. Infantile spasms are usually intractable, and prognosis is poor.
- Microdysgenesis, consisting of minor anomalies of cortical lamination and increased neurons in the white matter, has been proposed as a pathologic correlate in some cases of epilepsy but is still controversial.

TABLE 3.15 Developmental Cortical Malformations

I. Malformations due to abnormal neuronal and glial proliferation
A. Generalized
1. Decreased proliferation: microencephaly
a. Thin cortex
b. Normal cortex
2. Increased proliferation: none known
3. Abnormal proliferation (abnormal cell types): none known; probably not compatible with survival
?Microgliomatosis
B. Focal or multifocal
1. Decreased proliferation: none known
2. Increased proliferation: none known
a. Hemimegalencephaly without balloon cells
3. Abnormal proliferation (abnormal cell types)
a. Non-neoplastic
Tuberous sclerosis, types 1 and 2
Focal cortical dysplasia with balloon cells
Hemimega/encephaly with balloon cells
Isolated
In neurocutaneous syndromes
Epidermal nevus syndrome
Hypomelanosis of Ito
Klippel-Trenaunay syndrome
Focal transmantle dysplasia
b. Neoplastic
Dysembryoplastic neuroepithelial tumor
Ganglioglioma
Gangliocytoma
II. Malformations due to abnormal neuronal migration
A. Generalized
1. Classic (type 1) lissencephaly
a. Chromosome 17-linked
Miller-Dieker syndrome*
Isolated lissencephaly sequence*
b. X-linked
X-linked lissencephaly*
Subcortical band heterotopias*
c. Other loci
Isolated lissencephaly sequence
Other syndromes
2. Cobblestone (type 2) lissencephalies
a. Fukuyama-type congenital muscular dystrophy
b. Walker-Warburg syndrome*
c. Muscle-eye-brain disease*
3. Lissencephaly: not otherwise classified
4. Pachygyria
5. Unlayered polymicrogyria

TABLE 3.15 *Continued*

6. Heterotopia
    a. Subependymal
        X-linked (bilateral periventricular nodular heterotopia)
        Sporadic
    b. Subcortical
    c. Subpial
7. Cortical infoldings (symmetric)

B. Focal or multifocal
1. Focal agyria/pachygyria (partial lissencephaly)
    a. Bilateral posterior pachygyria
    b. Bilateral parietal pachygyria
2. Unlayered polymicrogyria
3. Focal or multifocal heterotopia
    a. Focal subependymal nodular
    b. Focal subcortical nodular
    c. Focal mixed subcortical/subependymal
    d. Focal subpial
        Fetal alcohol syndrome
        Other
4. Cortical infoldings (unilateral)
5. Focal or multifocal heterotopias with overlying organizational abnormality of the cortex
    a. Focal subependymal nodular
    b. Focal subcortical nodular
    c. Focal mixed subcortical/subependymal
        Aicardi syndrome
        Peroxisomal disorders
    d. Cortical infoldings (unilateral or asymmetric)
    e. Focal subpial
6. Excessive single ectopic white matter neurons

III. Malformations due to abnormal cortical organization

A. Generalized
1. Polymicrogyria (PMG), classic

B. Focal or multifocal
1. PMG
    a. Bilateral symmetric PMG
        Bilateral frontal PMG
        Bilateral perisylvian PMG
        Bilateral occipital PMG
    b. Asymmetric PMG (same as 1a)
2. Schizencephaly and mixed schizencephaly/PMG
3. Focal or multifocal cortical dysplasia without balloon cells
4. Microdysgenesis

IV. Developmental cortical malformations, not otherwise classified

*Allelic or possibly allelic.

Source: Reprinted with permission from RI Kuzniecky, AJ Barkovich. Pathogenesis and pathology of focal malformations of cortical development and epilepsy. J Clin Neurophysiol 1996;13:469–470.

- Other developmental/congenital conditions associated with epilepsy:
  - Schizencephaly
  - Porencephaly (see Figure 4.20)
  - Subarachnoid cyst (see Figure 4.21)

Mesial Temporal Sclerosis

- Mesial temporal sclerosis is the most common pathologic finding in patients undergoing temporal lobectomy for temporal lobe epilepsy (Van Paesschen, 1997). It is found in approximately 40% of resected specimens for intractable temporal lobe epilepsy.
- The pathology involves a variable degree of neuronal loss and gliosis, especially in the CA1 and CA3 fields; the dentate gyrus and hilum may show similar changes. MRI shows evidence of mesial temporal sclerosis (hippocampal atrophy, increased signal, and disruption of internal architecture), especially with volumetric analysis, in approximately 50% of cases with intractable temporal lobe epilepsy (see Figure 4.31). The amygdala may be affected as well.
- May occur bilaterally.
- "Dual pathology" (i.e., concurrent cortical or subcortical dysplasias, vascular malformations or tumors) may occur.
- The etiologies of mesial temporal sclerosis are likely multiple, with prolonged febrile convulsions in childhood most often identified.

Porphyria

- Seizures, usually generalized tonic-clonic, can occur in hepatic porphyrias during acute attacks and, less frequently, between attacks.
- Attacks may be iatrogenically induced (e.g., by barbiturates or sulfonamides).
- High carbohydrate intake and hematin are used to treat acute attacks and to reduce porphyrin excretion.
- The traditional AEDs—barbiturates, phenytoin, carbamazepine, valproate, and benzodiazepines—have all been found to induce porphyrin production to a greater or lesser degree and therefore should be avoided.
- Bromides have been used to treat seizures in porphyria, and vigabatrin and gabapentin have been found not to induce porphyrin production and could be used. Of the newer agents, lamotrigine has been found to induce porphyrin production.

Alcohol

- Five percent to 15% of persons with alcoholism experience seizures, which are related to withdrawal in two of three cases.
- More than 20% of newly diagnosed adult epilepsy patients have no risk factors other than alcoholism.
- Alcohol withdrawal seizures ("rum fits")
  - Usually with chronic, heavy alcohol use, but may occur after only weeks of heavy drinking.

  - Follow abrupt cessation of drinking or reduction of high alcohol intake.
  - Most common interval between cessation of drinking and seizures is 18–24 hours; 90% of seizures occur between 7 and 48 hours postcessation.
  - Affected individuals most commonly have two to four seizures within 6 hours.
  - Sixty percent have multiple seizures and 3% status epilepticus.
  - Thirty percent develop delirium tremens.
- Alcoholism is associated with a threefold increased risk for seizures.
- Heavy alcohol use appears to be an independent, dose-related risk factor for seizures apart from withdrawal seizures. Part of this risk may be due to a concurrent increased risk for head injury.
- Alcohol is also a specific provoking factor for seizures in some epileptic patients. In addition, alcohol use may result in low AED levels in epileptic patients due to poor compliance, reduced absorption, and hepatic enzyme induction.

Drugs

The drugs listed in Table 3.16 may provoke seizures or lower the seizure threshold in epileptic patients. Many of them cause seizures, particularly with overdose.

Head Trauma

- *Early* seizures are designated as those occurring in the first week after head injury, versus late post-traumatic seizures or epilepsy. The incidence of early seizures following closed head injury was 9.4% in children younger than 5 years, 3.3% in children between 6 and 15 years of age, 5.1% in those ages 16–25 years, 4.1% in adults ages 26–45 years, and 1.5% in adults ages 46–65 years (Jennett and Lewin, 1960). Early seizures occurred in 2.6% of children (<15 years old) and in 1.8% of adults following closed head injury (Annegers et al., 1980), but were much more common with severe closed head injury (30.5% in children and 10.3% in adults).
- In Jennett's series (1979) of hospitalized head injury patients, the presence of early seizures increased the risk of late epilepsy from 3% to 25% and was more important in patients older than 15 years old.
- The overall risk of late post-traumatic epilepsy varies from 9% to 42% in civilian population head injuries series, and from approximately 40% to 50% in military penetrating head injuries (Brain Trauma Foundation, 1996; Jennett, 1979).
- Risk of late epilepsy following missile injuries to the head is increased if there is an intracranial hematoma, dural penetration, or brain laceration (Table 3.17).
- Fifty-seven percent of those with late-onset epilepsy (>1 week postinjury) develop it within 1 year of injury, 85% within 2 years, and almost all by 5 years.
- Although epilepsy is rare as a consequence of mild head injury, it can occur, possibly due to small cortical or intracerebral hemorrhages.

TABLE 3.16 Some Drugs That May Provoke Seizures

	Relatively Commonly	*Occasionally or Rarely*
Therapeutic agents	Penicillin (high dose, renal failure, cardiac bypass); isoniazid (especially overdose); aminophylline; theophylline; tricyclic antidepressants (especially overdose); phenothiazines; clozapine; insulin/oral hypoglycemics; antihistamines	Lidocaine and other local anesthetics (IV); general anesthetics; cycloserine; antimalarials; cyclosporine; meperidine; fentanyl; morphine; radiographic contrast agents (meglumine derivatives, metrizamide); ceftazidime; metronidazole; tacrine; acyclovir; beta-blockers; lithium; bupropion; interferon-α, 4-aminopyridine
Drugs of abuse (recreational)	Cocaine; amphetamine/methamphetamine; cannabis (overdose); lysergic acid diethylamide; phencyclidine hydrochloride	—
Withdrawal seizures	Benzodiazepines; barbiturates; other antiepileptic drugs; amphetamines; opiates; baclofen	Allopurinol

- EEG adds little to the prediction of post-traumatic epilepsy (Jennett, 1979).
- A population-based Mayo Clinic retrospective/prospective study (Annegers et al., 1998) followed 4,541 head injury patients (38% pediatric), largely untreated with AEDs, for more than 10 years. It divided cases according to severity, as shown in Table 3.18. Standardized incidence ratios (i.e., compared to the general population) for late, unprovoked seizures were calculated and related to head injury severity. Ratios for seizures following mild, moderate, and severe head injuries were 1.5 (not significantly increased), 2.9, and 17.0. The probability of having at least one seizure in the first 5 years in these three groups was 0.7%, 1.2%, and 10%, respectively. The most significant risk factors for late seizures were brain contusion, subdural hematoma, and, to a lesser degree, loss of consciousness or amnesia after 24 hours or if the patient was older than 65. Early seizures did not influence the probability of late seizures.
- Neither phenytoin nor carbamazepine reduces the incidence of late post-traumatic seizures. In 1996, the Brain Trauma Foundation recommended that

TABLE 3.17 Factors Influencing the Risk of Late Post-Traumatic Epilepsy after Closed Head Injury

Depressed skull fracture	17%
>24 hrs post-traumatic amnesia	32%
<24 hrs post-traumatic amnesia	9%
No depressed skull fracture	3%
Early seizures (in first week)	25%
No early seizures	3%
Intracranial hematoma requiring surgical therapy	35%
No intracranial hematoma	3%
No depressed fracture, hematoma, early seizures or prolonged (>24 hrs) post-traumatic amnesia	<1%

Source: WB Jennett. Epilepsy after Non-Missile Head Injuries (2nd ed). London: Heinemann Medical Books, 1975.

they could, however, be used in the first week postinjury to prevent early seizures in high-risk patients.

Acquired Immunodeficiency Syndrome

- In one series, new-onset seizures were seen in 13% of 630 acquired immunodeficiency syndrome (AIDS) patients (Wong et al., 1990).
- Most of the cerebral pathologies that can affect human immunodeficiency virus (HIV) patients can produce seizures, including HIV encephalopathy, toxoplasmosis (see Figure 4.22), cerebral lymphoma, cryptococcal meningitis, and cerebral infarction. In addition, seizures may be related to illicit drug use, alcohol withdrawal, or electrolyte disturbances.
- In patients with low CD4 counts, opportunistic infection is the most likely cause and may be the initial symptom. Most seizures occur late in the course of the illness, but early seizures can occur in HIV-positive patients who have no symptoms of AIDS.
- Investigations should include drug toxicology screen, EEG, neuroimaging and cerebrospinal fluid (CSF) examination.
- Unless an identifiable, reversible cause is found, maintenance AED therapy should be initiated because of a high rate of recurrence, even after a single seizure, in AIDS patients.

Other Infectious or Immunologic Conditions

- Three percent of *bacterial meningitis* survivors develop epilepsy, and 10% of those with acute seizures develop epilepsy.

TABLE 3.18 Risk of Post-Traumatic Epilepsy (PTE) and Severity of Head Injury

Severity of Head Injury	*Late PTE[a] at 1 yr*	*Late PTE at 5 yrs*
Mild closed head injury (no skull fracture and <30 mins unconsciousness or amnesia)	0.1%[b]	0.6%[b]
Moderate (nondepressed skull fracture or unconsciousness or amnesia >30 mins but <24 hrs)	0.7%	1.6%
Severe (intracranial hematoma, cerebral contusion or unconsciousness or amnesia >24 hrs)	7.1% (10% with early seizures in adults, 30% in children)	11.5%

[a]Late epilepsy is defined as one or more seizures occurring after the first week post-trauma.

[b]Not increased versus general population.

Source: JF Annegers, JD Grabow, RV Groover, et al. Seizures after head trauma: a population study. Neurology 1980;30:683–689.

- *Cerebral abscesses*, particularly in frontal and temporal regions, may lead to epilepsy in up to 72% of surviving patients. Tuberculosis is a common cause of brain abscess in developing countries and has a high tendency to cause seizures.
- Between 10% and 25% of survivors of *herpes simplex encephalitis* develop epilepsy, the higher figure applying to patients having seizures during acute illness.
- Cerebral *cysticercosis* is an important cause of epilepsy in Mexico, South America, India, and Africa. The larval form of the tapeworm *Taenia solium* infests the brain, causing multiple cystic lesions that calcify later (see Figure 4.23).
- Epilepsy is relatively frequent in *Creutzfeldt-Jakob disease*, a transmissible spongiform encephalopathy due to prions. Myoclonus is often most prominent.

Cerebral Tumors

- Approximately 40% of adults presenting with new partial-onset epilepsy have a cerebral tumor.
- Ten percent to 30% of patients with chronic intractable partial epilepsy harbor low-grade neoplasms, usually in the medial temporal areas (see Figure 4.33).
- Slow-growing tumors, such as meningiomas or low-grade gliomas, are more likely to present with epilepsy than are rapidly growing tumors, such as glioblastomas (see Figure 4.34).

- Gangliogliomas (see Figure 4.32) and dysembryoplastic neuroepithelial tumors (DNETs) are found primarily in the medial temporal areas and are overrepresented in patients with epilepsy. They are slow-growing, almost hamartomatous lesions with neuronal and glial elements. Gangliogliomas may occasionally become cystic and grow rapidly.
- A 1993 report from Morris et al. shows that a long history of epilepsy and normal neurologic examination do not rule out an underlying tumor such as a slow-growing oligodendroglioma, ganglioglioma, or DNET as a cause.
- A 1998 report from the same group showed that, despite long-term, medically resistant epilepsy, a good outcome can be expected following surgical excision of gangliogliomas.
- A specific type of gelastic (laughing) seizure has been associated with and is virtually pathognomonic of hypothalamic hamartoma (Berkovic et al., 1988). These seizures often begin in early childhood and consist of short outbursts of forced, mechanical, mirthless laughter with or without impairment of consciousness. Seizures are frequent, may be accompanied by other seizure types including complex partial seizures, and are often resistant to treatment. Patients may also develop cognitive impairment and behavioral problems. Temporal lobe surgery is not helpful in most cases.

Multiple Sclerosis

- Seizures occur in up to 5–10% of cases at some time during the illness, due to impingement of plaques on cortical gray matter.
- In a population-based study conducted by Engelsen and Gronning (1997), the prevalence of epilepsy was 3.8% in 423 multiple sclerosis (MS) patients. Seizures began at a mean of 7 years after onset of MS.
- Seizures may be partial or, more frequently, secondarily generalized.
- Painful tonic spasms are a type of paroxysmal event, possibly arising from basal ganglia, which is seen almost exclusively in MS and which responds to AEDs.
- Status epilepticus or a series of severe convulsive seizures may cause a permanent deterioration of neurologic status.

Cerebrovascular Disease

- Stroke is the most common cause of late-onset epilepsy (after age 50), accounting for 50–80% of cases.
- MRI has revealed occult cerebral ischemic lesions as a cause for late-onset epilepsy in an increasing number of patients and is much more sensitive than CT for detecting small (especially mesial temporal) ischemic lesions (see Figure 4.35).
- Seizures occur acutely (within 2 weeks) in approximately 8% of patients with a carotid territory infarction or supratentorial intracerebral hemorrhage and are significantly more common in the latter (Kilpatrick et al., 1990).
- Epilepsy or seizures occur in approximately 40% of cases of large arteriovenous malformations and are relatively common in cavernous hemangiomas (see Fig-

ure 4.36). Multiple cavernous hemangiomas (see Figure 4.37) may occur as part of a familial syndrome with autosomal dominant inheritance.

- Rarely berry aneurysms can cause epilepsy without obvious subarachnoid hemorrhage (see Figure 4.24).
- Epilepsy (late recurrent seizures) occurs in 5–10% of cerebral infarcts and in 2.5–25.0% of cerebral hemorrhages. Most of the epilepsy develops within the first 2 years poststroke.
- Cortical infarction, especially following middle cerebral artery occlusion, is most likely to lead to seizures or epilepsy. The size of infarct, whether the infarct is thrombotic or embolic, and the EEG in the acute phases were not significant risk factors in most series.
- Other factors that increase the likelihood of late-developing epilepsy following stroke are the occurrence of early seizures (in the first 1–2 weeks poststroke) in most series and possibly the degree of residual neurologic deficit.
- A 1996 community-based prospective study conducted by So et al. from the Mayo Clinic followed 535 infarcts (90% supratentorial) for a mean of 5.5 years. Six percent (33 of 535) had early seizures, 78% in the first 24 hours. Embolic and anterior hemisphere infarcts were significantly associated with early seizures. Six percent (27 of 436) of survivors developed late seizures, representing a risk of 8–9% by 10 years poststroke, or six times the risk in the general population; 4.1% (18 of 27) developed epilepsy. Early poststroke seizures and recurrent strokes were predictive of epilepsy; embolic strokes or results of EEG when performed acutely were not.
- Seizures or epilepsy are more common following cerebral infarcts or intracerebral hemorrhage in childhood than in adulthood. The incidence of seizures is 19% (16% epilepsy) following infarction and 29% (26% epilepsy) following hemorrhage (Kluger et al., 1996).

Cerebral Degenerative Disease

- Up to 14% of late-onset seizures are due to *Alzheimer's disease*.
- Seizures occur in approximately 15% of patients with Alzheimer's disease surviving 10 years, usually late in the course. The seizures are usually mild, but generally are associated with a poor prognosis of the Alzheimer's disease.
- Alzheimer's patients with myoclonus seem to have an increased risk of seizures.
- Epilepsy is frequent in *chorea with acanthocytosis*.

Suggested Reading

Differential Diagnosis

Aldrich MS. Sleep related spells associated with parasomnias and narcolepsy. Semin Neurol 1995;15:194–201.

Bleasel A, Kotagal P. Paroxysmal nonepileptic disorders in children and adolescents. Semin Neurol 1995;15:203–215.

Chabolla DR, Krahn LE, So EL, et al. Psychogenic nonepileptic seizures. Mayo Clinic Proc 1996;1:493-500.

Devinsky O, Sanchez-Villasenor F, Vazquez B, et al. Clinical profile of patients with epileptic and nonepileptic seizures. Neurology 1996;46:1530-1533.

Fisher RS. Imitators of Epilepsy. New York: Demos Publications, 1994.

Kuyk J, Leijten F, Meinardi H, et al. The diagnosis of psychogenic nonepileptic seizures: a review. Seizure 1997;6:243-253.

Lagerlund TD, Cascino GD, Cicora KM, Sharbrough FW. Long-term electroencephalographic monitoring for diagnosis and management of seizures. Mayo Clinic Proc 1996;71: 1000-1006.

Leis AA, Ross MA, Summers AK. Psychogenic seizures: ictal characteristics and diagnostic pitfalls. Neurology 1992;42:95-99.

Lesser RP. Psychogenic seizures. Neurology 1996;46:1499-1507.

Levitan M, Bruni J. Repetitive pseudoseizures incorrectly managed as status epilepticus. Can Med Assoc J 1986;134:1029-1031.

Mahowald MW, Schenck CH. NREM sleep parasomnias. Neurol Clin 1996;14:675-696.

Morrell MJ. Differential diagnosis of seizures. Neurol Clin 1996;11:737-754.

Murphy JV, Dehkharghani F. Diagnosis of childhood seizure disorders. Epilepsia 1994; 35(Suppl 2):S7-S12.

Pacia SV, Devinsky O, Luciano DJ, Vazquez B. The prolonged QT syndrome presenting as epilepsy: a report of two cases and literature review. Neurology 1994;44:1408-1410.

Pedley TA. Differential diagnosis of episodic symptoms. Epilepsia 1983;24(Suppl 1):S31-S44.

Riley TL, Roy A (eds). Pseudoseizures. Baltimore: Williams & Wilkins, 1982.

Schenck CH, Mahowald MW. REM sleep parasomnias. Neurol Clin 1996;14:697-696.

Classification of Seizures and Syndromes

Aicardi J. Syndromic classification in the management of childhood epilepsy. J Child Neurol 1994;9(Suppl 2):S14-S18.

Andermann F, Zifkin B. The benign occipital epilepsies of childhood: an overview of the idiopathic syndromes and of the relationship to migraine. Epilepsia 1998;39(Suppl 4): S9-S23.

Andrews PI, Dichter MA, Berkovic SF, et al. Plasmapheresis in Rasmussen's encephalitis. Neurology 1996;46:242-246.

Antel JP, Rasmussen T. Rasmussen's encephalitis and the new hat. Neurology 1996;46:9-11.

Benbadis SR, Luders HO. Epileptic syndromes: an underutilized concept. Epilepsia 1996;37:1029-1034.

Berkovic S, Andermann F, Andermann E, Gloor P. Concepts of absence epilepsies: discrete syndromes or biological continuum? Neurology 1987;37:993-1000.

Christie S, Guberman A, Tansley BW, Couture M. Primary reading epilepsy: investigation of critical seizure-provoking stimuli. Epilepsia 1988;29:288-293.

Commission on Classification and Terminology of the International League Against Epilepsy. Proposal for revised clinical and electroencephalographic classification of epileptic seizures. Epilepsia 1981;22:489-501.

Commission on Classification and Terminology of the International League Against Epilepsy. Proposal for a revised classification of epilepsies and epileptic syndromes. Epilepsia 1989;30:389-399.

Commission on Pediatric Epilepsy of the International League Against Epilepsy. Myoclonus and epilepsy in childhood. Epilepsia 1997;38:1251-1254.

Dreifuss FE. Malignant Syndromes of Childhood Epilepsy. In RJ Porter, D Chadwick (eds), The Epilepsies 2. Boston: Butterworth-Heinemann, 1997;157-165.
Duchowny M, Harvey M. Pediatric epilepsy syndromes: an update and critical review. Epilepsia 1996;37(Suppl 1):S26-S40.
Dulac O. Epileptic syndromes in infancy and childhood: recent advances. Epilepsia 1995;36 (Suppl 1):S51-S57.
Dulac O. Benign Syndromes in Childhood Epilepsy. In RJ Porter, D Chadwick (eds), The Epilepsies 2. Boston: Butterworth-Heinemann, 1997;167-186.
Forster FM. Reflex Epilepsy, Behavioral Therapy and Conditional Reflexes. Springfield, IL: Charles C. Thomas, 1977.
French JA, Williamson PD, Thadani VM, et al. Characteristics of medial temporal lobe epilepsy: 1. Results of history and physical examination. Ann Neurol 1993;34:774-780.
Gobbi G, Sorrenti G, Santucci M, et al. Epilepsy with bilateral occipital calcifications: a benign onset with progressive severity. Neurology 1988;38:913-920.
Gordon N. The Landau-Kleffner syndrome: increased understanding. Brain Dev 1997;19: 311-316.
Holmes GL. Neonatal seizures. Sem Pediatr Neurol 1994;1:72-82.
Janz D. Juvenile myoclonic epilepsy: epilepsy with impulsive petit mal. Cleve Clin J Med 1989;56(Suppl 1):S23-S33.
Jay V, Becker LE, Otsubo H, et al. Chronic encephalitis and epilepsy (Rasmussen's encephalitis). Neurology 1995;45:108-117.
Kotagal P, Arankumar GS. Lateral frontal lobe seizures. Epilepsia 1998;39(Suppl 4):S62-S68.
Kuzniecky R. Symptomatic occipital lobe epilepsy. Epilepsia 1998;39(Suppl 4):S24-S31.
Laskowitz DT, Sperling MR, French JA, et al. The syndrome of frontal lobe epilepsy. Neurology 1995;45:780-787.
Lea ME, Harbord M, Sage MR. Bilateral occipital calcification associated with celiac disease, folate deficiency and epilepsy. AJNR 1995;16:1498-1500.
Lerman P, Kivity S. The benign partial nonrolandic epilepsies. J Neurophysiol 1991;8: 275-287.
Luciano D. Partial seizures of frontal and temporal origin. Neurol Clin 1996;11:805-822.
Lüders H, Lesser RP (eds). Epilepsy: Electroclinical Syndromes. London: Springer-Verlag, 1987.
Marseille Consensus Group. Classification of progressive myoclonic epilepsies and related disorders. Ann Neurol 1990;28:113-116.
Panayiotopoulos CP, Obeid T, Tahan AR. Juvenile myoclonic epilepsy: a 5 year prospective study. Epilepsia 1994;35:285-296.
Porter RJ. The absence epilepsies. Epilepsia 1993;34(Suppl 3):S42-S48.
Rasmussen T, Andermann F. Update on the syndrome of "chronic encephalitis" and epilepsy. Cleve Clin J Med 1989;56(Suppl 2):S181-S184.
Riggio S. Frontal lobe epilepsy: clinical syndromes and presurgical evaluation. J Epilepsy 1995;8:178-189.
Ritaccio AL. Reflex seizures. Neurol Clin 1994;12:57-83.
Roger J, Bureau M, Dravet C, et al. Epileptic Syndromes in Infancy, Childhood and Adolescence. Paris: John Libbey, 1992.
So NK. Mesial frontal epilepsy. Epilepsia 1998;39(Suppl 4):S49-S61.
Tiacci C. Epilepsy with bilateral occipital calcifications: Sturge-Weber variant or a different encephalopathy? Epilepsia 1993;34:528-539.
Vining EP, Freeman JM, Brandt J, et al. Progressive unilateral encephalopathy of childhood (Rasmussen's syndrome): a reappraisal. Epilepsia 1993;34:639-650.
Wheless JW, Constantinu EC. Lennox-Gastaut syndrome. Pediatr Neurol 1997;17:203-212.

Williamson PD, French JA, Thadani VM, et al. Characteristics of medial temporal lobe epilepsy: 2. Interictal and ictal scalp electroencephalography, neuropsychological testing, neuroimaging, surgical results and pathology. Ann Neurol 1993;34:781-787.

Wirrell EC. Benign epilepsy of childhood with centrotemporal spikes. Epilepsia 1998;39 (Suppl 4):S32-S41.

Zifkin B, Andermann F (eds). Reflex Epilepsies and Reflex Seizures. Advances in Neurology. Vol. 75. Philadelphia: Lippincott-Raven, 1997.

Febrile Seizures

Baumann RJ, D'Angelo SL. Technical report summary: the neurodiagnostic evaluation of the child with a first febrile seizure. Pediatrics 1996;97:773-775.

Berg AT, Shinnar S. Unprovoked seizures in children with febrile seizures—short term outcome. Neurology 1996;47:562-568.

Berg AT, Shinnar S, Darefsky AS, et al. Predictors of recurrent febrile seizures. A prospective cohort study. Arch Ped Adolesc Med 1997;151:371-378.

Bergman DA, Baltz RD, Cooley JR, et al. Practice parameter: the neurodiagnostic evaluation of the child with a first febrile seizure. Pediatrics 1996;97:769-772.

Camfield PR, Camfield CS. Management and treatment of febrile seizures. Curr Probl Pediatr 1997;27:6-14.

Camfield P, Camfield C, Gordon K, et al. What types of epilepsy are preceded by febrile seizures? A population based study of children. Dev Med Child Neurol 1994;36:887-892.

Maher J, McLachlan RS. Febrile convulsions in selected large families: a single-major-locus mode of inheritance? Dev Med Child Neurol 1997;39:79-84.

Nelson KB, Ellenberg JH. Prognosis in children with febrile seizures. Pediatrics 1978;61: 720-727.

Nelson KB, Ellenberg JH. Prenatal and perinatal antecedents of febrile seizures. Ann Neurol 1990;27:127-131.

Rosman NP. Therapeutic options in the management of febrile seizures. CNS Drugs 1997;7:26-36.

Rosman NT, Colton T, Labazzo J, et al. A controlled trial of diazepam administered during febrile illnesses to prevent recurrent febrile seizures. N Engl J Med 1993;329:79-84.

Sceffer IE, Berkovic SF. Generalized epilepsy with febrile seizures plus: a genetic disorder with heterogeneous clinical phenotypes. Brain 1997;120:479-490.

Verity CM. Febrile Convulsions: A Pragmatic Approach. In RJ Porter, D Chadwick (eds), The Epilepsies 2. Boston: Butterworth-Heinemann, 1997;289-311.

Verity CM, Greenwood R, Golding J. Long term intellectual and behavioral outcomes of children with febrile convulsions. N Engl J Med 1998;338:1723-1728.

Etiology of Epilepsy

Ambrosetto G, Antonini L, Tassinari C. Occipital lobe seizures related to clinically asymptomatic celiac disease in adulthood. Epilepsia 1992;33:476-481.

Annegers JF, Grabow JD, Groover RV, et al. Seizures after head trauma: a population study. Neurology 1980;30:683-689.

Annegers JF, Hauser WA, Coan SP, et al. A population-based study of seizures after traumatic brain injuries. N Engl J Med 1998;338:20-24.

Asconapé JJ, Penry JK. Poststroke seizures in the elderly. Clin Geriatr Med 1991;7:483-492.

Barkovich AJ. Malformations of neocortical development: magnetic resonance imaging correlates. Curr Opin Neurol 1996;9:118-121.

Barkovich AJ, Peacock W. Sublobar dysplasia. A new malformation of cortical development. Neurology 1998;50:1383–1387.

Berkovic SF, Andermann F, Melanson D, et al. Hypothalamic hamartomas and ictal laughter: evolution of a characteristic epileptic syndrome and diagnostic value of magnetic resonance imaging. Ann Neurol 1988;23:429–439.

Bernasconi A, Bernasconi N, Andermann F, et al. Celiac disease, bilateral occipital calcifications and intractable epilepsy: mechanisms of seizure origin. Epilepsia 1998;39:300–306.

Brain Trauma Foundation. The role of antiseizure prophylaxis following head injury. J Neurotrauma 1996;11:731–734.

Cendes F, Cok MJ, Watson C, et al. Frequency and characteristics of dual pathology in patients with lesional epilepsy. Neurology 1995;45:2058–2064.

Clark GD, Fishman MA. Neuronal Migration Disorders and Epilepsy. In SH Appel (ed), Current Neurology. Amsterdam: IOS Press 1997;17:237–264.

Cohen BH. Metabolic and degenerative diseases associated with epilepsy. Epilepsia 1993; 34(Suppl 3):S62–S70.

Engelsen BA, Gronning M. Epileptic seizures in patients with multiple sclerosis. Is the prognosis of epilepsy underestimated? Seizure 1997;6:377–382.

Giroud MGP, Gras P, Fayolle N, et al. Early seizures after acute stroke: a study of 1,640 cases. Epilepsia 1994;35:959–964.

Guberman A, Jaworski ZFG. Pseudohypoparathyroidism and epilepsy: diagnostic value of computerized cranial tomography. Epilepsia 1979;20:541–553.

Holtzman DM, Kaku DA, So YT. New onset seizures associated with human immunodeficiency virus infection: causation and clinical features in 150 cases. Am J Med 1989;87: 173–177.

Jennett B. Post-traumatic epilepsy. Adv Neurol 1979;22:137–147.

Jennett B, Lewin W. Traumatic epilepsy after closed head injuries. J Neurol Neurosurg Psychiatr 1960;23:295–301.

Jennett WB. Epilepsy after Non-Missile Head Injuries (2nd ed). London: Heinemann Medical Books, 1975.

Kilpatrick CJ, Davis SM, Hopper JL, et al. Early seizures after acute stroke: risk of late seizures. Arch Neurol 1992;49:509–511.

Kilpatrick CJ, Davis SM, Tress BM, et al. Epileptic seizures in acute stroke. Arch Neurol 1990;47:157–160.

Kinnunen E, Wikstrom J. Prevalence and prognosis of epilepsy in patients with multiple sclerosis. Epilepsia 1986;27:729–733.

Kotagol P, Rothner AD. Epilepsy in the setting of neurocutaneous syndromes. Epilepsia 1993;34(Suppl 3):S71–S78.

Kuzniecky RAF, Guerrini R. Congenital bilateral perisylvian syndrome: study of 31 patients. The CBPS Multicenter Study. Lancet 1993;341:608–612.

Lee N, Radtke RA, Gray L, et al. Neuronal migration disorders: positron emission tomography correlations. Ann Neurol 1994;35:290–297.

Mahteiro L, Nunes B, Mendonca D, et al. Spectrum of epilepsy in neurocysticercosis: a long-term follow-up of 143 patients. Acta Neurol Scand 1995;92:33–40.

Moots P, Maciunas RJ, Eisert DR. The course of seizure disorders in patients with malignant gliomas. Arch Neurol 1995;51:717–724.

Morris HH, Estes ML, Gilmore R, et al. Chronic intractable epilepsy as the only symptom of primary brain tumor. Epilepsia 1993;34:1038–1043.

Morris HH, Matkovic Z, Estes ML, et al. Ganglioma and intractable epilepsy: clinical and neurophysiologic features and predictors of outcome after surgery. Epilepsia 1998;39:307–313.

Pringle CE, Blume WT, Munox DG, et al. Pathogenesis of mesial temporal sclerosis. Can J Neurol Sci 1993;20:184–193.

Raymond AA, Fish DR, Sisodiya SM, et al. Abnormalities of gyration, heterotopias, tuberous sclerosis, focal cortical dysplasia, microdysgenesis, dysembryoplastic neuroepithelial tumour and dysgenesis of the archicortex in epilepsy. Clinical EEG and neuroimaging features in 100 adult patients. Brain 1995;118:629–660.

Raymond AA, Fish DR, Stevens JM, et al. Association of hippocampal sclerosis with cortical dysgenesis in patients with epilepsy. Neurology 1994;44:1841–1845.

Raymond AA, Fish DR, Stevens JM, et al. Subependymal heterotopia: a distinct neuronal migration disorder associated with epilepsy. J Neurol Neurosurg Psychiat 1994;57: 1195–1202.

Sander JWAS, Hart YM, Johnson AL, et al. The National General Practice Study of Epilepsy: newly diagnosed seizures in a general population. Lancet 1990;336:1267–1271.

Sloviter RS. The functional organization of the hippocampal dentate gyrus and its relevance to the pathogenesis of temporal lobe epilepsy. Ann Neurol 1994;35:640–654.

So EL, Annegers JF, Hauser WA, et al. Population-based study of seizure disorders after cerebral infarction. Neurology 1996;46:350–355.

Swanson TH. The pathophysiology of human mesial temporal lobe epilepsy. J Clin Neurophys 1995;12:2–22.

Thompson AJ, Kermode AG, Moseley IF, et al. Seizures due to multiple sclerosis: seven patients with MRI correlations. J Neurol Neurosurg Psychiatr 1993;56:1317–1320.

Van Paesschen W. Quantitative MRI of mesial temporal structures in temporal lobe epilepsy. Epilepsia 1997;38(Suppl 10):3–12.

Wong MC, Suite NDA, Labar DR. Seizures in human immunodeficiency virus infection. Arch Neurol 1990;47:640–642.

Zentner JWH, Ostertun B. Gangliogliomas: clinical, radiological and histopathological findings in 51 patients. J Neurol Neurosurg Psychiatry 1994;57:1497–1502.

Genetics of Epilepsy

Charlier C, Singh NA, Ryan SG, et al. A pure mutation in a novel KQT-like potassium channel gene in an idiopathic epilepsy family. Nat Genet 1998;18:53–55.

Delgado-Escueta A, Greenberg D, Weissbecker K, et al. Gene mapping in the idiopathic generalized epilepsies: juvenile myoclonic epilepsy, childhood absence epilepsy, epilepsy with grand mal seizures and early childhood myoclonic epilepsy. Epilepsia 1990;31 (Suppl 3):S19–S29.

Dobyns WB, Andermann E, Andermann F. X-linked malformations of neuronal migration. Neurology 1996;47:331–339.

Elmslie S, Gardiner RM. Epilepsy and the New Genetics. In RJ Porter, D Chadwick (eds), The Epilepsies 2. Boston: Butterworth-Heinemann, 1997;49–70.

Gedda L, Tatarelli R. Essential isochronic epilepsy in MZ twin pairs. Acta Genet Med Gemellol (Roma) 1971;20:380–383.

Greenberg DA, Durner M, Resor S, et al. The genetics of idiopathic generalized epilepsies of adolescent onset. Neurology 1995;45:942–946.

Serratosa JM, Delgado-Escueta AV, Medina MT, et al. Clinical and genetic analysis of a large pedigree with juvenile myoclonic epilepsy. Ann Neurol 1996;39:187–195.

Treiman LJ. Genetics of epilepsy: an overview. Epilepsia 1993;34(Suppl 3):S1–S11.

4 Investigations

Metabolic Screening

- In certain syndromes, especially those occurring in childhood, with a family history, or with a progressive course or those accompanied by other unexplained neurologic deficits, screening for inherited and occasionally acquired metabolic abnormalities is necessary. Some of the metabolic tests are listed in Table 4.1; others are a logical extension of the discussion of etiologies in Chapter 3.
- The tests listed in Table 4.1 are useful in screening for the underlying etiology in selected cases of epilepsy, particularly when no etiology is clearly evident from the history and examination, when the epilepsy or seizures are localization-related (apart from benign rolandic and other benign epilepsies of childhood), or when neurologic abnormalities or myoclonus accompanies the epilepsy.

Electroencephalography

Technique

- EEG was first used in humans by Hans Berger in 1924 (the first report of its use was published in 1929).
- An EEG is a tracing of voltage fluctuations versus time recorded from electrodes placed over the scalp in a specific array. These microvolt voltages represent fluctuating dendritic potentials from superficial cortical layers and require amplification. Deep parts of the brain are not well sampled.
- The EEG tracing is a 20-minute or longer sampling of brain activity, which may be written out or recorded directly on magnetic tape or digitally by computer.
- Disc *electrodes* are applied according to the standard 10-20 system (Figure 4.1, Table 4.2). Extra electrodes may be added to increase spatial resolution, to record from specific areas, or to monitor other electrical activity (e.g., electro-oculographic monitoring; electrocardiographic [ECG] monitoring; nasopharyngeal or nasoethmoidal electrodes; infraorbital electrodes; zygomatic, minisphenoidal, or sphenoidal electrodes). Zygomatic electrodes for recording from mesial-temporal structures generally provide as much information as the other electrodes and are better tolerated.
- Various *montages* are used: reference (monopolar) run with an ear reference (not truly inactive), bipolar (e.g., double banana and coronal). With digital recordings, montages may be changed later for any section of the record.

TABLE 4.1 Tests to Consider in the Evaluation of Patients with Seizures

Seizure Type/ Syndrome	*Test*	*Comments*
Simple partial	MRI	Rule out structural lesion
Complex partial	MRI	Rule out structural lesion
Generalized tonic-clonic	MRI	Rule out structural lesion; most generalized seizures are secondarily generalized
Absences	None required	
Infantile spasms	Skin examination (Wood lamp)	Evaluate for hypopigmented macules (tuberous sclerosis)
	MRI	Useful for congenital malformations, including neuronal migrational abnormalities
	Amino acids, organic acids, biotinidase	Metabolic screening tests
	Ammonia (NH_3)	Useful for urea-cycle defects and other errors of metabolism
	Lactate/pyruvate	Useful screen for mitochondrial encephalopathies
	Pyridoxine infusion	Rule out vitamin B_6 dependency
	Ophthalmologic examination	Chorioretinitis may indicate congenital infection
Lennox-Gastaut	MRI	Rule out congenital anomaly
	Amino acids, organic acids, lysosomal enzymes	Useful screen for variety of metabolic disorders
	NH_3	Useful for screening for urea cycle defect and other errors of metabolism
	Serum lactate, pyruvate	Often abnormal in mitochondrial encephalopathy
	Ophthalmologic examination	Useful in ceroid lipofuscinosis
	Skin, rectal, conjunctival biopsy	Abnormal in ceroid lipofuscinosis
Progressive myoclonic epilepsy	MRI	Rule out congenital anomaly
	Lysosomal enzymes	Sialidosis, Gaucher's disease
	Skin biopsy	Useful in neuronal ceroid lipofuscinosis

Seizure Type/ Syndrome	Test	Comments
	Ophthalmologic examination	Useful in neuronal ceroid lipofuscinosis
	Muscle biopsy	Abnormal in mitochondrial disorders, Lafora's disease

MRI = magnetic resonance imaging.
Source: Reprinted with permission from G Holmes. In B Berg (ed), Principles of Child Neurology. New York: McGraw-Hill, 1996;254.

- Routine activation methods:
  - Eye opening and closure
  - Hyperventilation
  - Intermittent photic stimulation (2–60 Hz; eyes open, eyes closed and eye closure)
- Optional activation methods:
  - Sleep deprivation/sleep
  - Specific methods of seizure precipitation in some patients (e.g., video games, visual patterns)
  - AED withdrawal

Uses of Electroencephalography in Epilepsy

- To support diagnosis of epilepsy
- To help classify seizures
- To help localize the focus, especially in presurgical candidates
- To quantify seizures or epileptic bursts
- To aid in the decision of whether to stop AED treatment

TABLE 4.2 International 10-20 System of Electrode Placement

In 1958, the International System of Electrode Placement was established.
Electrodes are spaced at 10% or 20% of distances between specified anatomic landmarks.
Uses 21 electrodes, but others can be added.
Odd numbered electrodes over left hemisphere and even numbered over right hemisphere.

EEG is generally not a good guide to the effectiveness of treatment, except in certain instances (e.g., absence seizures with generalized spike-waves).

Advantages of Electroencephalography

- Is a measure of brain function and therefore supplements neuroimaging techniques
- Provides direct rather than indirect evidence of epileptic abnormality
- May be the only test technique that shows abnormalities in epileptic patients
- Provides some spatial or localization information
- Low cost
- Low morbidity
- Readily repeatable
- Portable/ambulatory

Disadvantages of Electroencephalography

- Relatively low sensitivity and specificity
- Subject to both electrical and physiologic artifacts
- Influenced by state of alertness, hypoglycemia, drugs
- Limited time sampling and spatial sampling

Specialized Electroencephalographic Techniques

- Intensive EEG/video monitoring (see the next section)
- Computerized analysis and brain electrical activity mapping (adds little to visual EEG interpretation in epilepsy)
- Magnetoencephalography:
  - Used at specialized centers to help localize epileptic foci (dipole localization) before epilepsy surgery
  - Very sensitive; can localize foci that are not localized by scalp EEG or MRI
  - Can be combined with MRI and PET to provide three-dimensional (3D) mapping of epileptiform activity
  - Very subject to electromagnetic field artifacts
  - Very expensive
- Polysomnography: useful for differentiating nocturnal, nonepileptic attacks, such as sleep apnea or parasomnias, from epileptic seizures

Intensive Electroencephalography/Video Monitoring for Epilepsy

Technique

- Cable or radiotelemetry and video; EEG and video recorded on videocassette, split-screen display.

- Ambulatory cassette monitoring (without video) can be used, especially in children who may have seizures in particular settings, such as at school.
- Inpatient (often presurgical) or outpatient laboratory.
- 8-hour versus continuous (inpatient). Several sessions are often necessary, and attempts should be made to record several spells.
- Intracranial electrodes (depth or subdural) for some presurgical patients.
- Automatic seizure detection and computerized data analysis can be used.
- Activation techniques to provoke seizures: hyperventilation, photic stimulation, drug withdrawal (caution with outpatients), sleep, specific stimuli (e.g., video games, reading) in reflex epilepsies.
- Tuning fork technique (or other noninvasive techniques) to provoke pseudoseizures: Patient is told, "We will apply a vibrating tuning fork to your forehead. This will send vibrations through your head and may provoke one of your spells so we can observe it." The technique can also be used at the bedside or in the clinic without EEG monitoring. To be a reliable indicator that the patient's attacks are pseudoseizures, the provoked attack should be similar to the patient's spontaneous spells. The similarity should be confirmed, if possible, by an observer who has seen the usual spells of the patient.
- Technologist must interact closely with the patient during the spell to accurately determine the degree of impairment of consciousness/amnesia.

Purpose

- To record seizures or spells or to obtain a prolonged interictal EEG sample
- To distinguish between epileptic seizures and other spells (e.g., pseudoseizures, syncope)
- To classify seizures (e.g., absence vs. complex partial)
- To localize the seizure focus, especially in epilepsy surgery candidates
- To quantify seizures when they occur frequently (e.g., absences)
- To make precise EEG/behavioral correlations

Electroencephalography Interpretation

- Waves are classified according to frequency (Hertz or cycles per second):
  1-3: delta
  4-7: theta
  8-13: alpha
  14-35: beta
- Amplitude is usually inversely related to frequency.
- *Background rhythms*: The predominant rhythm when the subject is relaxed with eyes closed. Usually a sinusoidal-appearing alpha rhythm in the posterior head regions. With eye-opening or arousal, it is replaced by a low-voltage, mixed-frequency (mainly beta) rhythm. Background rhythms are age-dependent, and theta or delta activity in posterior head regions is common in children.
- *Transients*: Stand out from background and are brief.

Abnormalities

- Slowing (intermittent or continuous):
  - Focal (suggests a lesion)
  - Generalized and background: drowsiness, postictal, metabolic, drugs, diffuse cerebral process
- Epileptiform features:
  - Interictal spikes, spike-waves, interictal paroxysmal rhythmic patterns
  - Ictal patterns
- Periodic (regular, recurring patterns)
- Hemispheric or lobar asymmetries

Activation Techniques

- *Hyperventilation* has a strong tendency to provoke generalized spike-wave discharges and bursts, especially in classic generalized "cortico-reticular" epilepsy. Focal spikes and various seizure types may also be triggered.
- *Slow-wave sleep* tends to exacerbate most epileptiform patterns, including spike-wave and focal spikes, and may change the morphology of the discharges.
- *Photoconvulsive response* (Figure 4.10) to intermittent photic stimulation shows frontal, central, and occipital spike-waves that are at a different frequency from the flash and that tend to outlast the duration of the flash. They must be distinguished from photomyoclonic responses, frontal electroretinal potentials, and normal, sharply contoured occipital driving responses. Only the true photoconvulsive response (one variety of photoparoxysmal response) correlates with photosensitive epilepsy.

Physiologic Electroencephalographic Activity That Can Be Confused with Epileptiform Activity

- *Vertex transients* of light sleep:
  - May occur in rhythmic bursts and be particularly sharp in young children (especially up to age 5).
  - Midline spikes (epileptic) may "ride" on the V waves.
  - May be asynchronous in young children.
- *Hypnagogic hypersynchrony*:
  - Appears in drowsiness, in first decade, especially before age 5
  - 3–5 Hz, high-amplitude bursts, maximal fronto-central, 1.5–3.0 seconds' duration
  - May be mistaken for spike-wave discharges when intermixed with fast activity
- *Positive occipital sharp transients of sleep* (POSTS) (Figure 4.2):
  - Occur in all stages of NREM sleep, particularly drowsiness and stage I
  - Occipital, may be asymmetric or unilateral, occur in short runs, at times 4–6 Hz

   - Have a sharp, lambdoid appearance
   - Can be mistaken for occipital sharp waves from an epileptic focus
- *Mu rhythm* (Figure 4.4):
   - Centro-temporal, 6- to 8-Hz rhythm
   - Rounded appearance with sharp phase
   - Blocked by contralateral fist clenching
- *Lambda waves*:
   - Occur in the occipital regions with visual scanning in some patients.
   - Sharp, lambdoid appearance may resemble epileptiform activity.
- *Breach rhythms* (Figure 4.6):
   - Sharp, high-frequency activity occurring over a skull defect (e.g., post-craniotomy).
   - High-frequency rhythms are normally attenuated by the intact skull.

Benign Epileptiform Variants of Unknown Clinical Significance

- Benign epileptiform transients of sleep:
   - Also known as *small sharp spikes*
   - Occur in one or both temporal regions (often independently) during light sleep
   - Occur individually, not in trains or bursts
   - Usually low-voltage with steep ascending phase and especially a steep descending phase when diphasic
   - May have a small after-coming slow wave
   - Fairly stereotyped in appearance, but may vary somewhat
   - Seen in adults 18 years of age and older
- 6- and 14-Hz positive spike bursts (Figure 4.5):
   - Mainly in children (peaks at age 13–14)
   - Seen mainly in drowsiness and light sleep
   - Positive spikes usually occur bilaterally, independently
   - Occur in bursts lasting less than 1 second
   - Most prominent in posterior temporal area
- Wicket spikes:
   - Mu-like rhythm in the temporal regions
   - Sharp bursts that are short and appear to be exaggerations of background rhythm
   - Occur predominantly in adults
   - In wakefulness and in sleep
- Occipital spike foci in children:
   - Less commonly associated with epilepsy than temporal or frontal spikes, and may disappear with age
   - May occur in children with early-onset visual deprivation
- Subclinical rhythmic EEG discharge of adults:
   - Mainly in elderly
   - Usually bilateral, posterior predominance

  - Begins with series of sharp-contoured waves that merge into a sustained, rhythmic theta frequency
  - May be superimposed on the background rhythm
- Rhythmic midtemporal theta discharge of drowsiness (rhythmic theta burst of drowsiness, psychomotor variant):
  - Trains of rhythmic, notched waves, 5–6 Hz
  - Usually bilateral
  - Invariable in form and frequency
  - Most prevalent in young adults
  - May last several minutes
  - Disappears with sleep
- Phantom spike-wave ("petit mal variant" of Gibbs):
  - 6 Hz
  - Low amplitude of spike
  - Predominates in adolescents and young adults
  - Seen during relaxed wakefulness and drowsiness; disappears during sleep
  - Short (usually 1–2 seconds), bisynchronous burst, maximal posteriorly or anteriorly

Electroencephalographic Findings in Epilepsy

- A normal EEG, even on repeated recordings, is found in 10–20% of epileptic patients. The likelihood of recording an abnormality depends partially on the number and length of recordings, the special electrodes used, the activation methods, and the type of epilepsy.
- Certain epilepsy syndromes have characteristics or suggestive features (Table 4.3).
- One percent to 2% of patients without a history of epilepsy show epileptiform features, especially spikes, on EEG. Between 5% and 45% of first-degree relatives of patients with primary generalized epilepsy had 3-Hz spike-wave bursts on their EEGs, despite being asymptomatic (Newmark and Penry, 1980). Patients with lesions such as tumors or strokes may show sharp activity without a history of seizure.
- The EEG must be interpreted in the light of its proximity to a seizure or seizures. Prolonged postictal slowing may occur in some cases.
- Background may be slowed by AEDs, underlying diffuse cerebral process, or postictal state.
- Artifact from eye rolling, tremor, other movement, electromyogram, electrodes, and other factors may resemble rhythmic ictal patterns. ECG, muscle spikes, movement, electrode popping, and other triggers may produce sharp activity resembling true epileptiform spikes or sharp waves.
- One of the difficulties of interpreting epileptiform activity is distinguishing between ictal and interictal bursts. Do prolonged epileptic paroxysms or even shorter bursts represent electrical seizures when there are no apparent behav-

TABLE 4.3 Seizure Disorders with Characteristic Electroencephalographic Features That May Aid in Diagnosis

Epilepsy syndromes	
Early infantile epileptic encephalopathy	Burst suppression
Early myoclonic encephalopathy	Burst suppression
Infantile spasms	Hypsarrhythmia
Childhood absence epilepsy	Generalized 3-Hz spike-wave
Juvenile myoclonic epilepsy	Generalized or multifocal 4–5 Hz spike-wave and polyspike-wave
Benign partial epilepsy with centrotemporal spikes	Unilateral or bilateral sharp-slow discharges with a horizontal dipole localizing to the central sulcus region
Benign occipital epilepsy	Unilateral or bilateral occipital sharp or sharp-slow activity that attenuates on eye opening
Landau-Kleffner syndrome	?Bilateral spike-wave activity with a horizontal dipole localizing to the superior temporal gyrus regions
Lennox-Gastaut syndrome	Generalized or bianterior spike-wave activity at <2.5 Hz
Neurologic disorders manifested by seizures with characteristic EEG features	
Alpers' syndrome	High-amplitude slow waves with superimposed multispikes
Subacute sclerosing panencephalitis	Periodic complexes
Neuronal ceroid lipofuscinosis	High-amplitude responses to slow photic stimulation
Angelman syndrome	Monomorphic rhythmic slowing of background
Lissencephaly	Augmentation of beta activity
Agenesis of the corpus callosum	Hemispheric asynchrony

Source: Reprinted with permission from M Duchowny, AS Harvey. Pediatric epilepsy syndromes: an update and critical review. Epilepsia 1996;37(Suppl 1):S28.

ioral accompaniments? In many cases, sensitive neuropsychological testing, such as determination of reaction time to a stimulus, reveals unsuspected behavioral accompaniments to paroxysmal spike-wave bursts as brief as 1–2 seconds. The interictal-ictal distinction is particularly difficult in patients with Lennox-Gastaut syndrome who may have prolonged or nearly continuous periods of slow spike-wave on the EEG.

Interictal Epileptiform Activity

- Sharp activity (Figures 4.7 and 4.8) appears over the epileptogenic area, but may also appear bilaterally, independently, or over more widespread areas and give false localizing information. Interictal spikes, spike-waves or sharp waves are seen bilaterally in 20–50% of patients with temporal lobe epilepsy.
- Interictal slowing or background asymmetries suggest a structural lesion.
- *Spikes*: 20–70 ms, pointed, stand out from background, diphasic or triphasic, usually surface negative, often followed by slow waves, have a reasonable field distribution.
- *Sharp-waves*: sharp theta transients, 70–200 ms; have the same significance as spikes.
- *Spike-waves*: single or multiple spikes followed by a theta or delta wave, generalized or focal:
  - Surface representation of paroxysmal depolarization shift in an aggregate of neurons.
  - Often occur in short bursts with varying frequency in the burst.
- Centro-temporal spikes of high amplitude, bilateral or unilateral, often triphasic, with a characteristic horizontal dipole; occur interictally in benign rolandic epilepsy of children.

Ictal Patterns

- A seizure has a beginning, an evolution, and an end and consists of rhythmic activity that stands out from the background.
- Ictal EEG is normal in greater than 60% of *simple partial seizures* but rarely with complex partial seizures.
- *Complex partial seizures* (Figure 4.14) almost invariably show rhythmic paroxysmal sharp theta activity, spike-waves, or slow waves that may spread bilaterally over one temporal or frontal-temporal area. Frontal complex partial seizures are not likely to be recorded by surface EEG or to show secondary bilateral synchrony. Low-voltage fast activity may precede rhythmic slow or sharp-slow activity in the areas from which the seizure originates.
- *Absence seizures* (Figures 4.11 and 4.12) show bilaterally synchronous rhythmic spike-waves or polyspike-waves, usually with a frequency of 2–4 Hz. Atypical absence attacks show spike-wave discharges that are either slower or faster than 3 Hz, have less clearly delineated spike-waves, may emerge more slowly from and return more gradually to normal background, and often have some interspersed slow waves.
- Some seizures, such as *tonic seizures* or *infantile spasms*, may show low-voltage fast activity diffusely (electrodecremental response).
- A *generalized tonic-clonic seizure* begins with an electrodecremental response (which may not be recorded from the scalp), followed by rhythmic

10-Hz spiking and then decelerating spike-wave discharges, followed by background flattening and slowing. The full pattern is not often apparent due to muscle artifact.

- *Epileptic myoclonus* may show spike-waves corresponding to the myoclonic jerks.
- *Generalized paroxysmal fast rhythms* are bursts of 15- to 25-Hz spikes (Figure 4.13) that are seen, particularly during sleep, in patients with multiple seizure types (e.g., Lennox-Gastaut).
- *Postictal EEG* may show slowing localized or lateralized to the site of seizure origin. Focal spikes tend to increase in frequency for hours or days following a partial seizure. Obtaining an EEG as soon as possible after a seizure may offer a better chance of localizing the site of seizure onset.

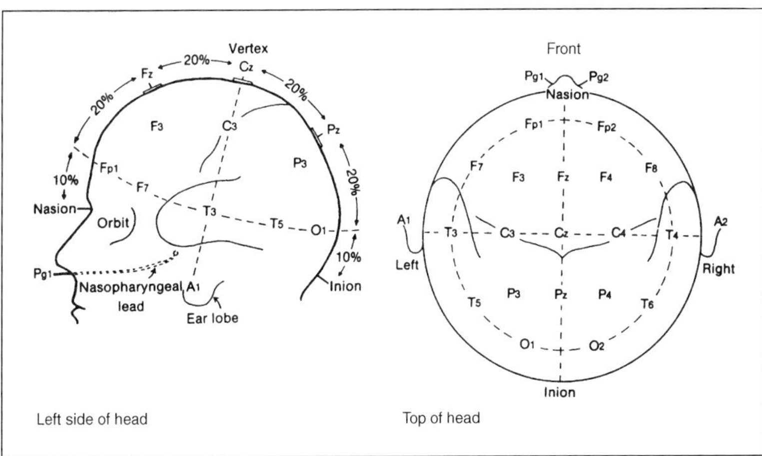

FIGURE 4.1 International 10-20 System of electrode placement for routine scalp electroencephalography.

Nonepileptiform Patterns That Could Be Mistaken for Epileptiform Abnormalities

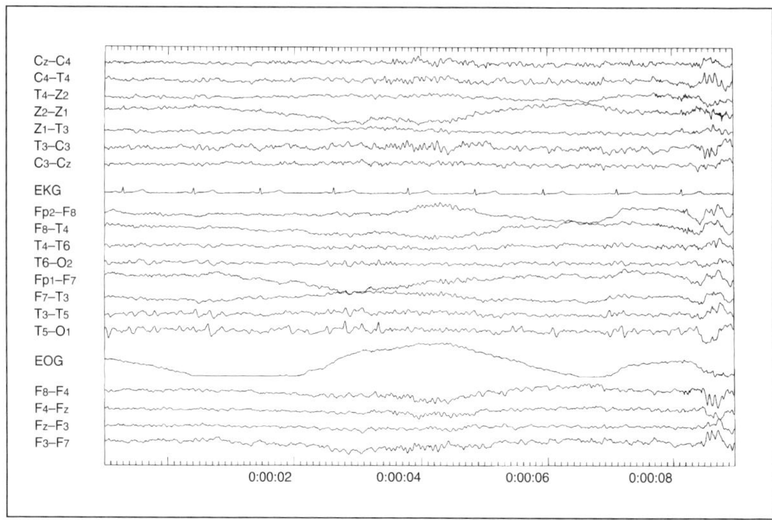

FIGURE 4.2 Asymmetric positive occipital sharp transients of sleep from left occipital region recorded during drowsiness in a 30-year-old man having spells of loss of consciousness.

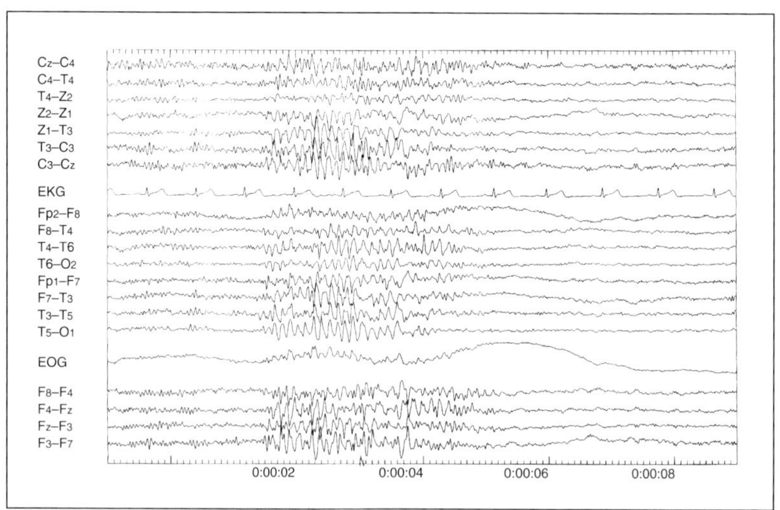

FIGURE 4.3 Theta burst of drowsiness (more prominent on the left) in a 30-year-old man with epilepsy since his teens.

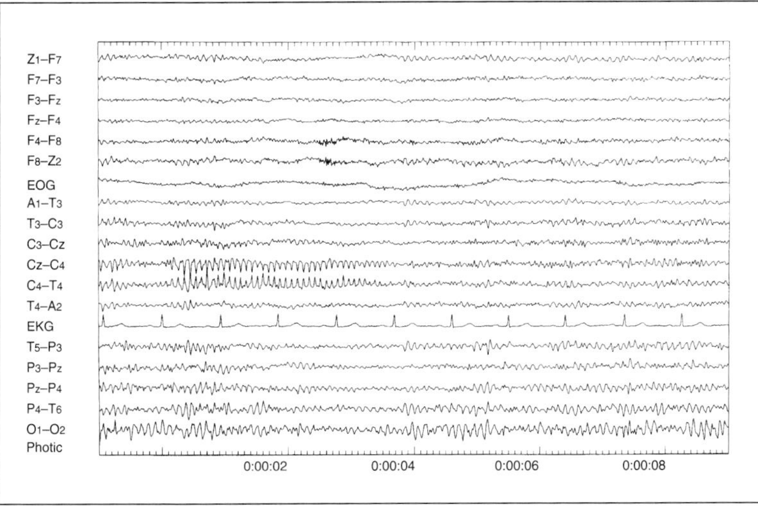

FIGURE 4.4 Asymmetric mu rhythm in a 59-year-old woman. The right central mu rhythm disappeared with clenching of the contralateral fist.

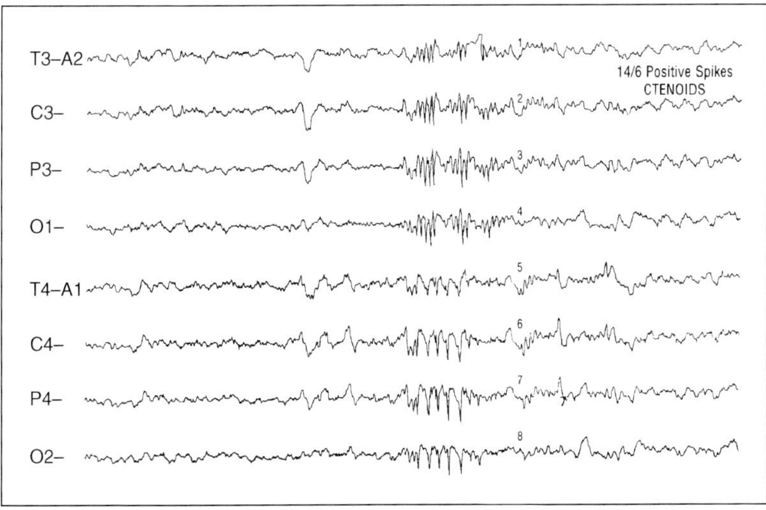

FIGURE 4.5 Fourteen- and 6-Hz positive spikes in a 33-year-old man with depression.

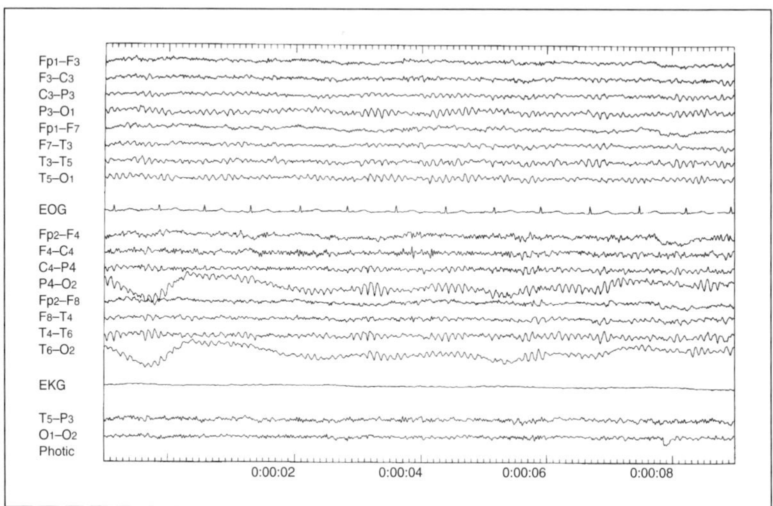

FIGURE 4.6 Breach rhythm over right fronto-centro-temporal area in a patient with previous right frontal craniotomy.

Interictal Abnormalities in Patients with Epilepsy

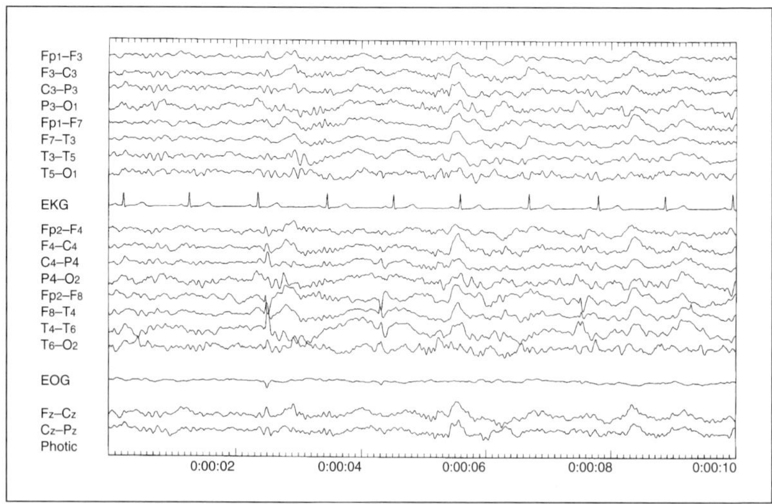

FIGURE 4.7 Right midtemporal sharp-wave focus in a patient with complex partial seizures.

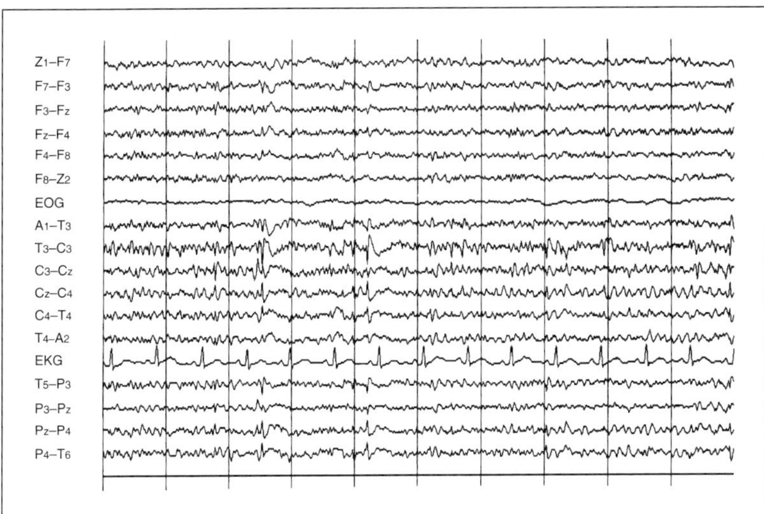

FIGURE 4.8 Left central spikes in a 28-year-old woman having repeated clonic seizures of the right arm.

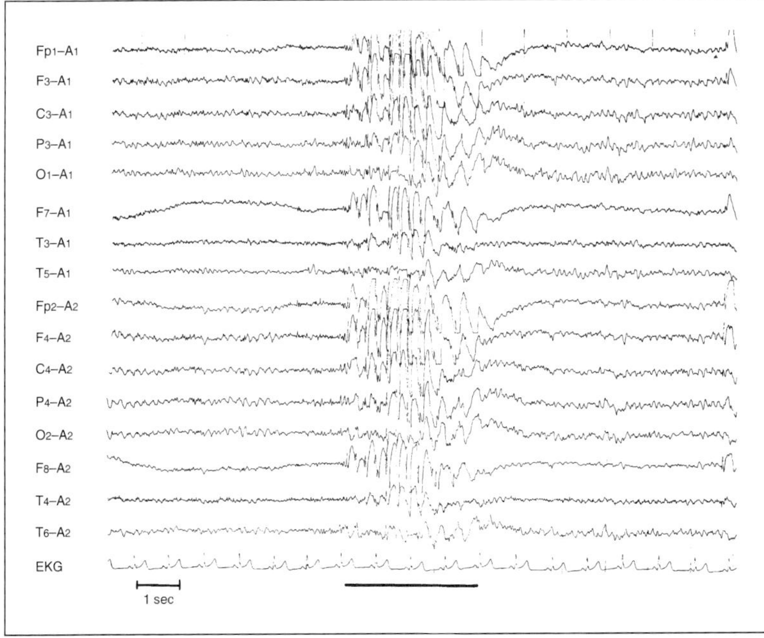

FIGURE 4.9 Generalized brief interictal spike-wave burst (marked by bar) in a 24-year-old woman with juvenile myoclonic epilepsy.

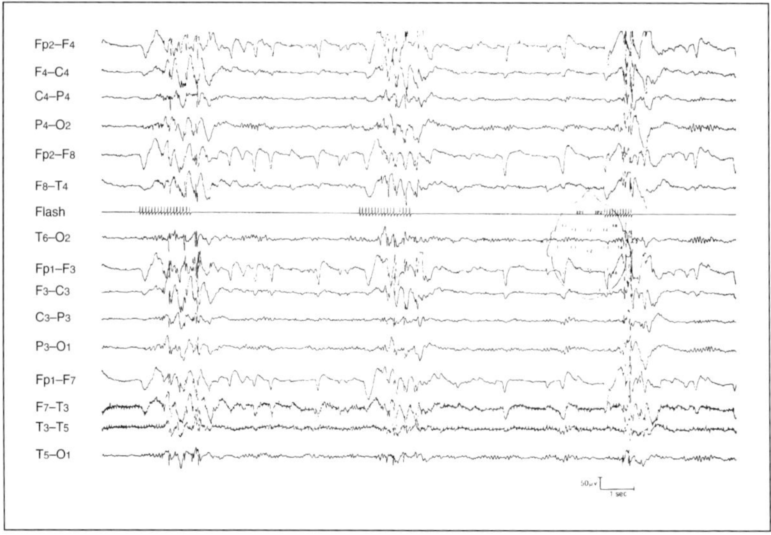

FIGURE 4.10 Photoparoxysmal response in an 18-year-old man with epilepsy. Flash is turned off when technologist notices buildup of generalized spike-wave. Note that the generalized discharges continue briefly after the flash.

Seizure Patterns

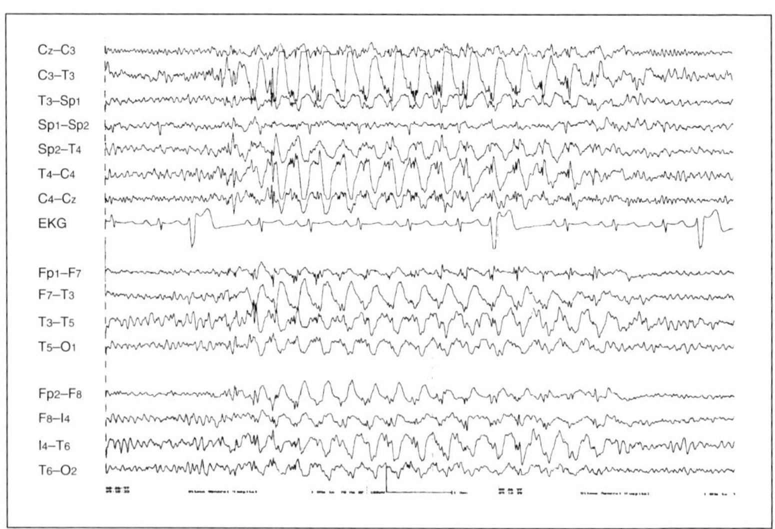

FIGURE 4.11 Brief absence seizure in an 18-year-old patient with primary generalized epilepsy.

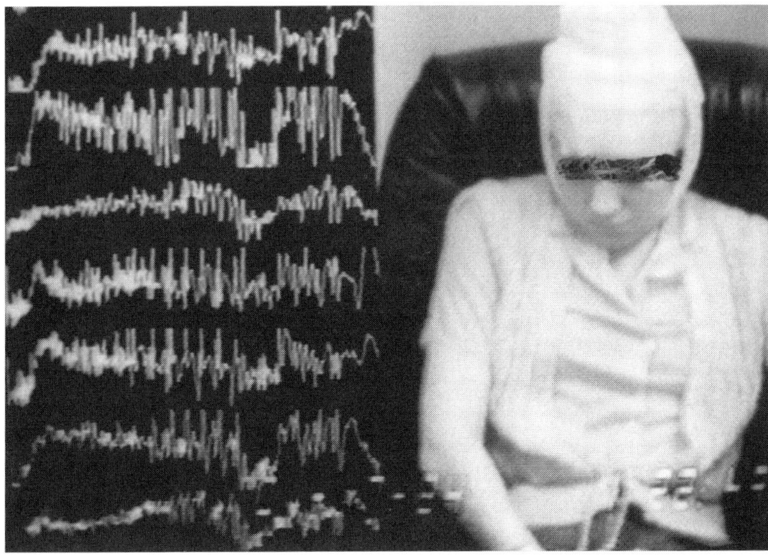

A

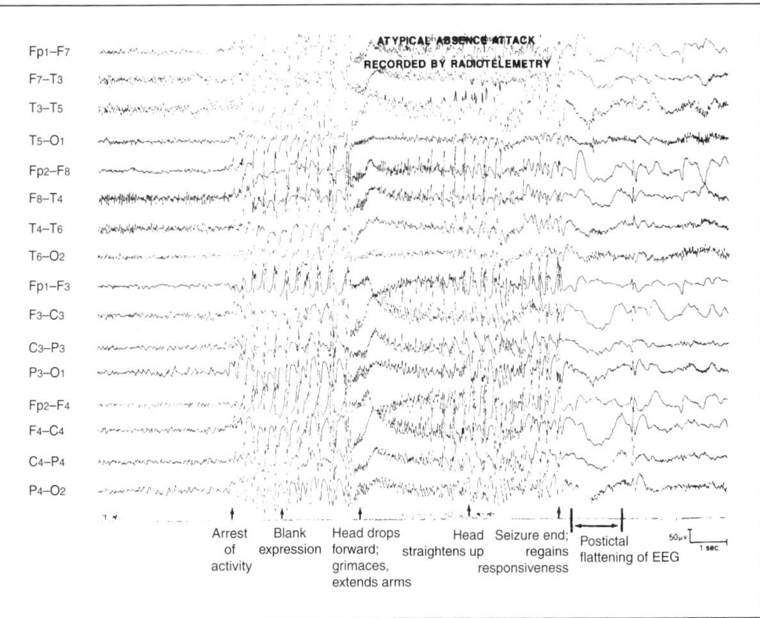

B

FIGURE 4.12 (**A**) Atypical absence attack in a 24-year-old woman recorded by electroencephalogram/video telemetry. (**B**) Note the correspondence between the electrical and behavioral events apparent upon analysis of the printed record in conjunction with the video.

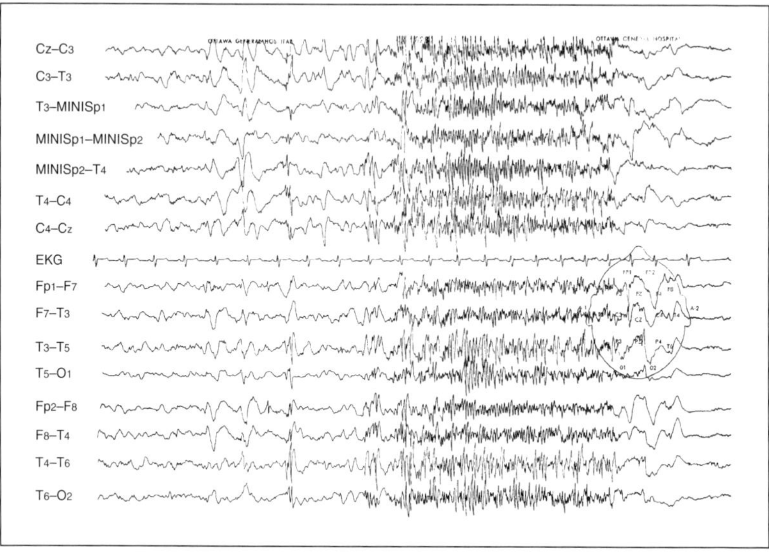

FIGURE 4.13 Patterns of a 24-year-old patient with Lennox-Gastaut syndrome. The electroencephalogram shows an atypical absence with tonic features beginning with generalized spike-wave followed by rapid generalized spiking and brief postictal background voltage suppression. Note the abnormal background.

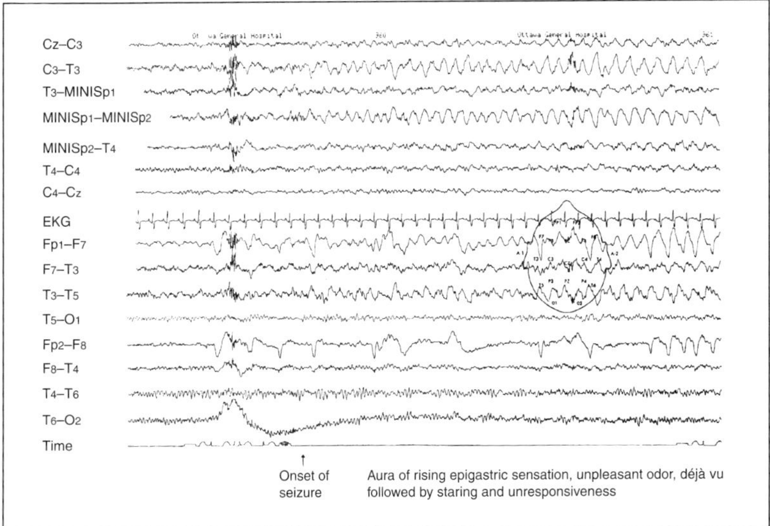

A

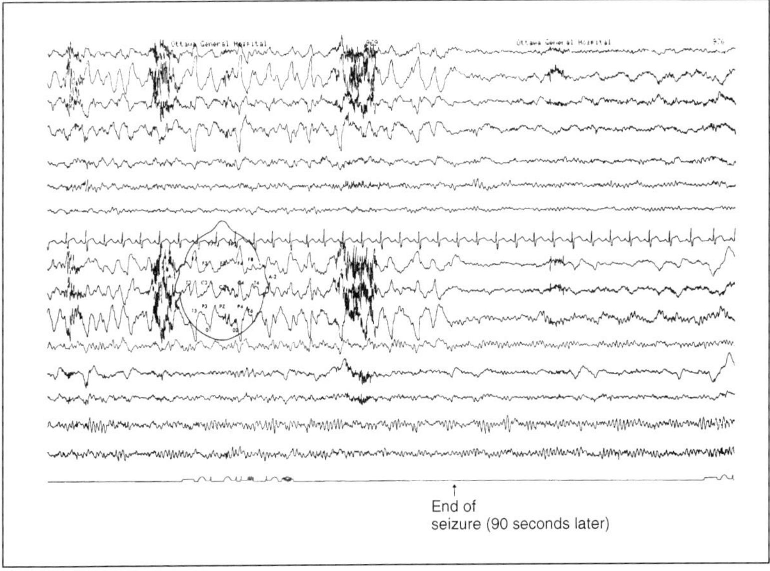

B

FIGURE 4.14 Left temporal complex partial seizure (only beginning [**A**] and end [**B**] shown) in a 20-year-old woman having olfactory auras and feelings of déjà vu during them. A left uncal low-grade astrocytoma was discovered on magnetic resonance imaging and successfully removed surgically.

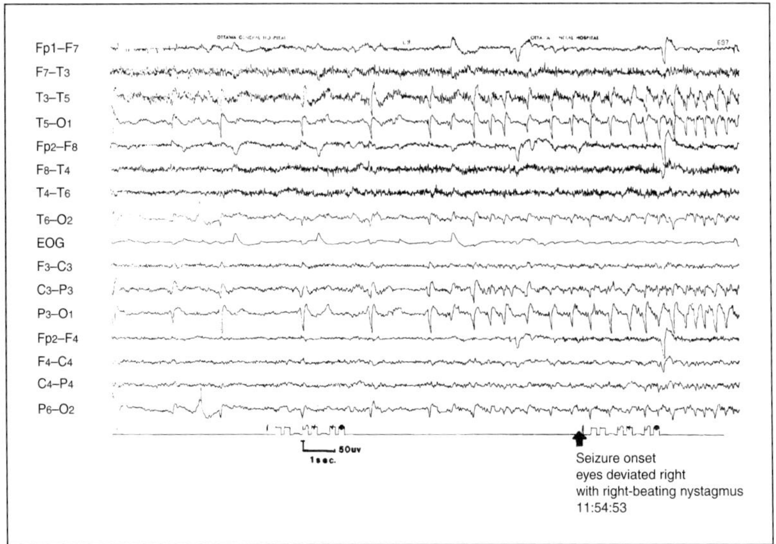

FIGURE 4.15 Left occipital status epilepticus in a 65-year-old woman manifested by contralateral conjugate eye deviation and nystagmus. Cause was not established.

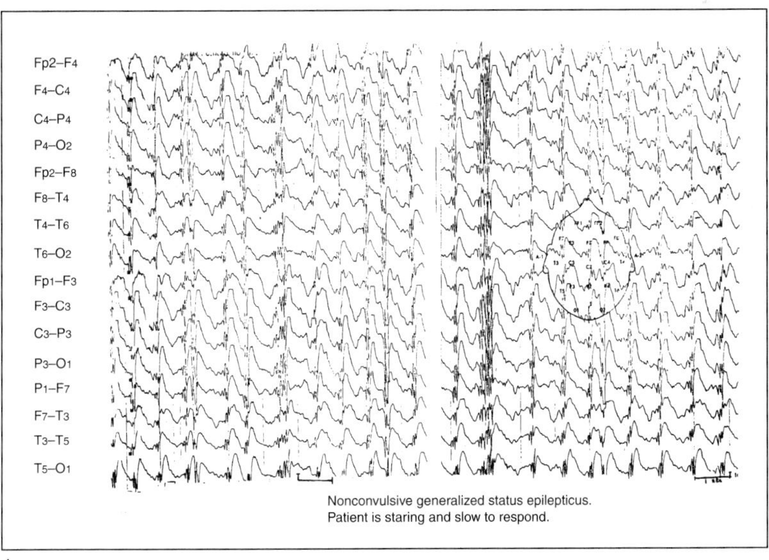

A

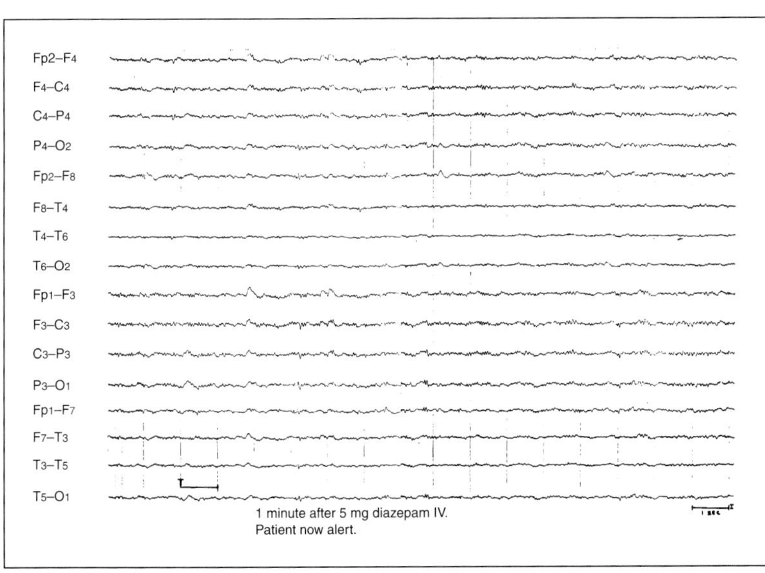

B

FIGURE 4.16 (**A**) Nonconvulsive generalized status epilepticus in a 17-year-old man. He was able to respond but appeared confused and had a long latency of response. (**B**) The second tracing shows return to alertness 1 minute after administration of intravenous diazepam.

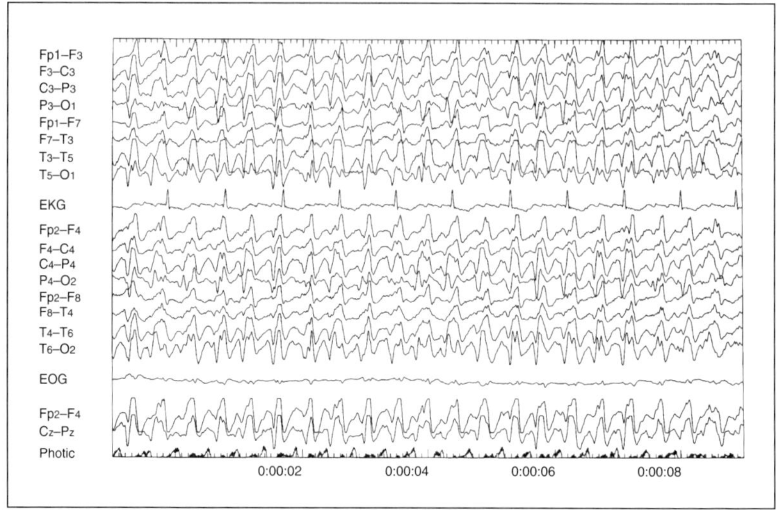

A

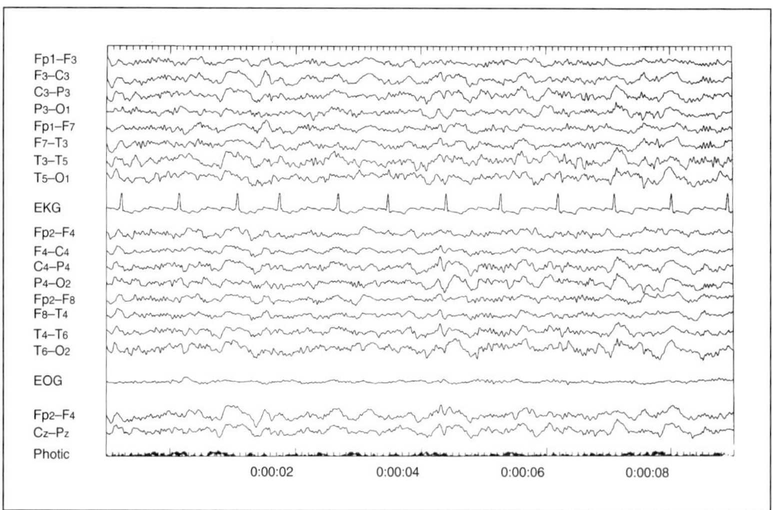

B

FIGURE 4.17 (**A**) A 76-year-old woman with long-standing multiple sclerosis presented with confusion and decreased responsiveness for 24 hours. Electroencephalogram (EEG) showed generalized nonconvulsive status epilepticus. (**B**) Two minutes after administration of intravenous lorazepam, 2 mg, the epileptic activity disappeared from the EEG. After sleeping, the patient was talking and responding as usual.

Neuroimaging

Indications

- All patients with epilepsy, except those with typical syndromes of primary generalized epilepsy (e.g., juvenile myoclonic epilepsy, childhood onset absences) or typical benign rolandic epilepsy, should have an initial CT or MRI.
- MRI is the procedure of choice and should be done when CT is negative, because it can detect abnormalities including subtle atrophies in the medial temporal regions, cortical gyral dysplasias, low-grade gliomas, and small cavernous hemangiomas, all of which may be missed on CT. Twelve percent to 30% of cases with a negative CT show relevant abnormalities on MRI.
- Even patients with long-standing epilepsy without known etiology should have neuroimaging. Oligodendroglioma or other tumors have been described in patients with histories of epilepsy longer than 20 years.
- In 1996, Greenberg et al. published guidelines for performing *emergency* neuroimaging studies in epilepsy patients. These guidelines are based on a review of the relevant literature:
  - Emergency scans (CT or MRI) should be performed on patients having *first-time seizures* with new focal neurologic deficits, persistent altered mental status (with or without intoxication), fever, recent head trauma, persistent headache, history of cancer, history of anticoagulation, or history or suspicion of AIDS. Partial seizures and age greater than 40 years are other possible indications for emergency neuroimaging studies in this group.
  - Emergency scans should be performed in patients with *known epilepsy* and recurrent seizures when there is a suspicion of a serious intracranial structural lesion on the basis of new focal deficits, persistent altered mental status (with or without intoxication), fever, recent head trauma, persistent headache, history of cancer, history of anticoagulation, or history or suspicion of AIDS. New seizure pattern or type and prolonged postictal confusion or worsening mental status are other possible indications.
- Neuroimaging, including MRI, magnetic resonance spectroscopy (MRS), 3D MRI, functional MRI (fMRI), and PET, has become an increasingly important part of the presurgical workup to identify epileptic foci in candidates for epilepsy surgery.
- Only when structural lesions correlate with the site of seizure origin, as determined by EEG studies and clinical analysis, can they be considered etiologically important. Dual pathology (e.g., tumor and mesial-temporal sclerosis) may be detected in some patients.

Computed Tomography

- CT has the advantage of being readily available and relatively cheap. It can detect sizable tumors, arteriovenous malformations (AVMs), major brain malformations, large strokes, and infectious lesions and is sensitive to calcified lesions and lesions of the skull. It is very insensitive to lesions at the base of the brain, in the orbitofrontal and mesial-temporal regions (partially due to the artifacts produced by bone), and small cortical lesions. Low-grade gliomas may be easily missed. Figures 4.18–4.24 show examples.

- CT is, however, useful when treating uncooperative patients, because scans can be obtained in seconds and are less susceptible to movement artifact than MRI is. It is useful in patients who cannot tolerate MRI or in whom MRI is contraindicated.
- If CT is done, contrast enhancement with coronal cuts is preferred for epileptic patients.

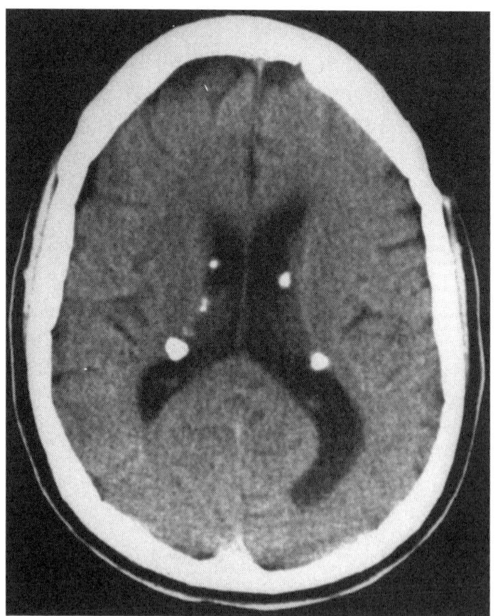

A

FIGURE 4.18 (**A**) Computed tomography showing typical subependymal calcified glial nodules in a 24-year-old man with tuberous sclerosis, severe mental retardation, marked adenoma sebaceum, and intractable seizures. (**B**) Numerous depigmented macules on his forearm, including one with an "ash-leaf" shape.

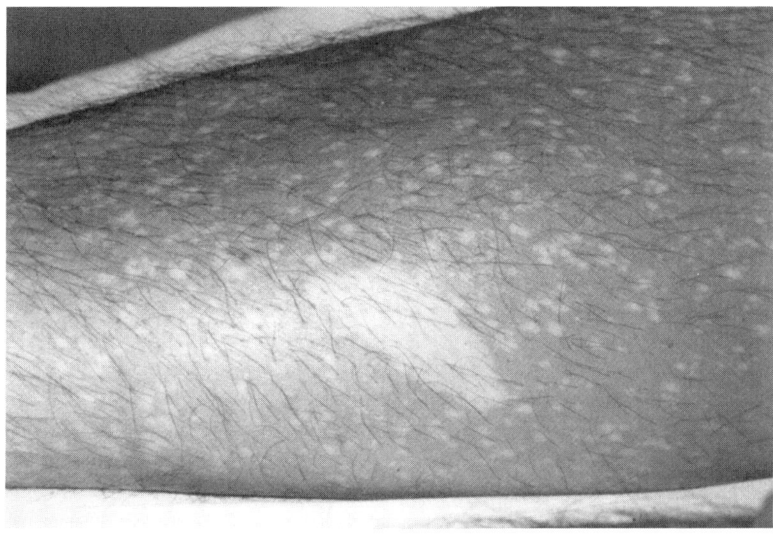

B

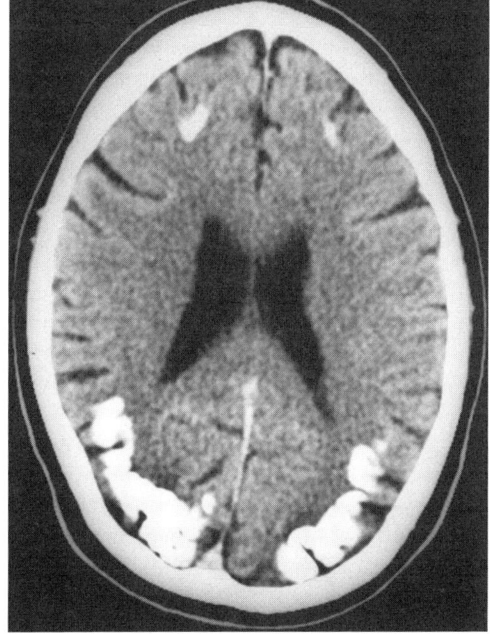

FIGURE 4.19 Computed tomography showing bioccipital and frontal calcifications in a 43-year-old man with partial seizures and a history of celiac disease in childhood.

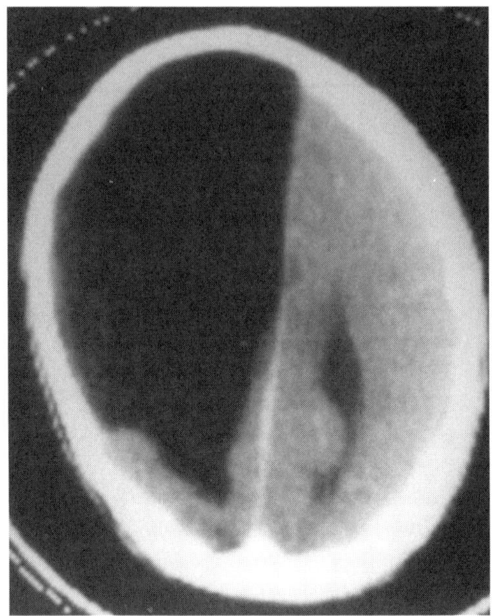

A

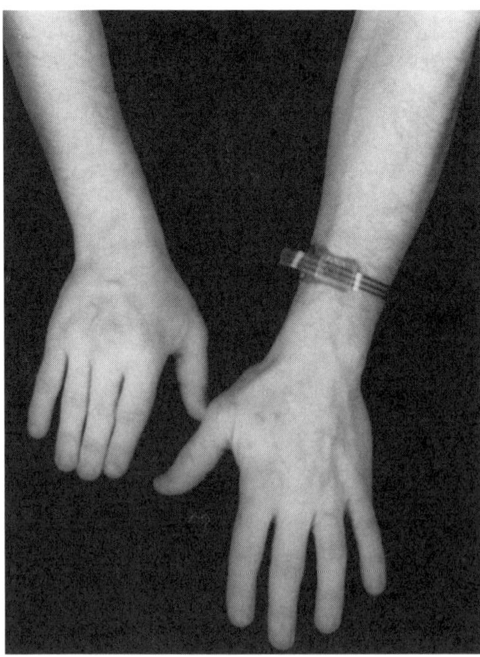

B

FIGURE 4.20 (**A**) Computed tomography showing massive porencephalic cyst in an 18-year-old man with infantile hemiplegia, hemiatrophy, and long-standing partial motor and secondarily generalized tonic-clonic seizures. (**B**) Hemiatrophy of the contralateral upper extremity.

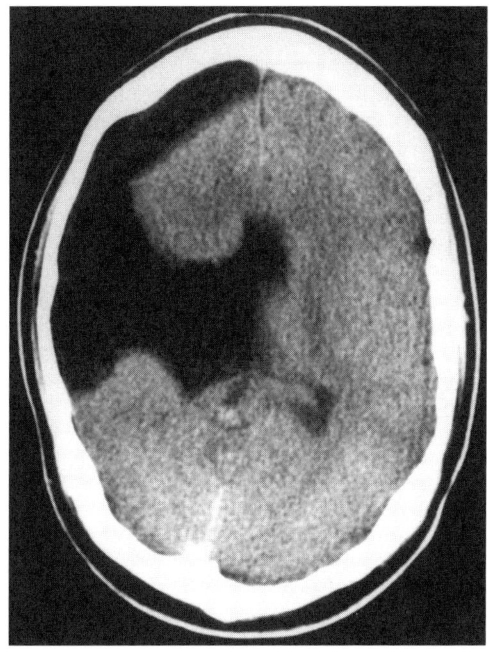

FIGURE 4.21 Computed tomography (CT) in an 18-year-old man with "cerebral palsy," epilepsy, and left hemiplegia. CT shows open-lipped right schizencephaly.

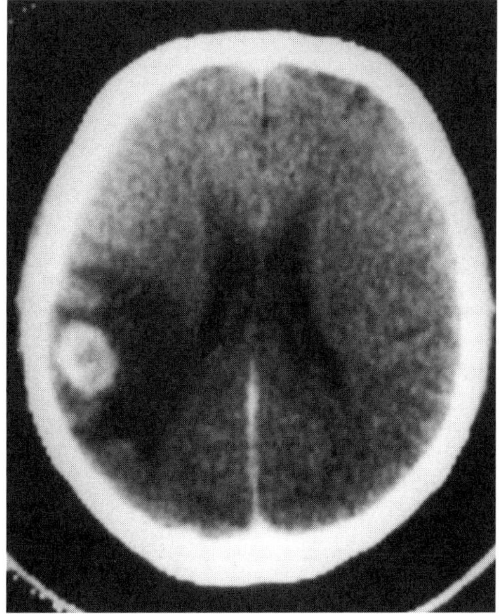

FIGURE 4.22 Computed tomography (CT) showing enhancing lesion with surrounding edema in a human immunodeficiency virus–positive man having a first seizure. CT suggests toxoplasmosis.

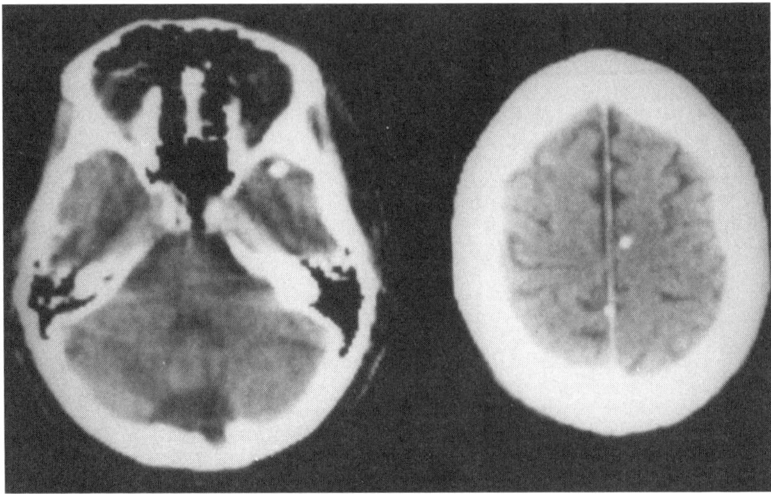

A

B

FIGURE 4.23 (**A**) Computed tomography in a 25-year-old patient with refractory complex partial seizures. Calcifications represent cysticercosis. (**B**) The resected specimen with the calcified lesion.

FIGURE 4.24 Computed tomography in a 54-year-old woman with a 6-week history of complex partial seizures. No headache or stiff neck was present. Three aneurysms are apparent around the circle of Willis. One is close to the right temporal lobe, where a seizure focus was recorded. Cerebrospinal fluid was clear. Angiography showed a right posterior communicating, left internal carotid, and basilar tip aneurysms. She died from a subarachnoid hemorrhage before surgery could be undertaken.

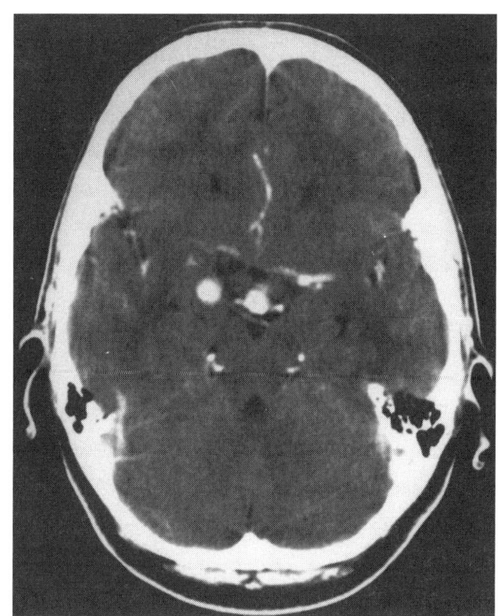

Magnetic Resonance Imaging

- Compared to CT, MRI produces superior spatial resolution, greater contrast between white and gray matter, better elimination of bone and soft tissue artifact, and much greater sensitivity to pathologic lesions that are isodense to brain tissue.
- MRI is the procedure of choice in epilepsy because of its sensitivity to features such as small lesions at the base of the brain, hippocampal atrophy, cortical dysplasias and neuronal migration abnormalities, low-grade and small gliomas, cavernous hemangiomas, and small subcortical ischemic areas (Figures 4.25–4.37).
- If thin contiguous slices are obtained, data can be reformatted in any plane, which compensates for asymmetric head positioning.
- Disadvantages: inability of some patients to tolerate the procedure due to claustrophobia; inability to perform the procedure without sedation in patients who are uncooperative; contraindications in patients with cardiac

pacemakers, ferromagnetic arterial clips, metallic skull plates, or intraocular metallic bodies; and relatively high cost of the procedure.

- The optimal technique is to use a 1.5-Tesla magnet and obtain both oblique coronal scans perpendicular to the hippocampus and oblique sections through the long axis of the hippocampus. Continuous cuts of 1.5 mm or less (for volume acquisition studies) are recommended.
- Gadolinium enhancement is rarely useful in the investigation of epileptic patients.
- T1- and T2-weighted scans are done routinely in coronal and sagittal planes. T1-weighted scans permit good differentiation between gray and white matter.
- The MRI protocol should be individualized for each patient according to the type of epilepsy and the suspected underlying pathology. For example, when looking for developmental anomalies, Kuzniecky and Jackson (1995) recommended the following sequence:
  - Screening images with intermediate contrast sequence
  - T1-weighted midline sagittal plane
  - T1-weighted thin coronal slices (1.0–1.5 mm) through the whole brain, providing volume 3D acquisitions that can be reformatted in three planes
  - Coronal inversion recovery sequences
- Features of hippocampal sclerosis on MRI (Figure 4.26) (Jackson, 1994):
  - Unilateral atrophy (including dilatation of temporal horn)
  - Loss of internal architecture on inversion recovery images
  - Increased signal on T2-weighted images
  - Decreased signal on T1-weighted images
- In a small proportion of cases of hippocampal sclerosis, signal change can occur in the absence of atrophy.
- Volumetric analysis allows a quantitative assessment of unilateral hippocampal atrophy and its anterior-posterior distribution, which can be useful for presurgical workup. This quantitative approach is more sensitive than visual inspection. Unilateral hippocampal atrophy correlates well with mesial-temporal sclerosis and predicts a good surgical outcome.
- T2 relaxometry is a method of quantifying abnormal tissue characteristics, is more sensitive than standard techniques, and allows determination of bilateral hippocampal abnormalities. Normal T2 relaxation times in the hippocampus are 99–106 ms.
- 3D reconstructions provide a detailed view of gyration abnormalities, which can be missed by routine studies. Sisodiya et al. (1996) found such abnormalities in the frontal lobes of 7 of 16 partial epilepsy patients whose routine imaging studies were negative.

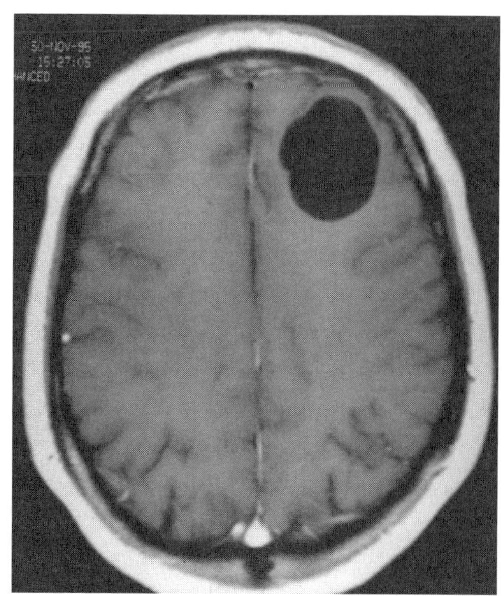

FIGURE 4.25 Magnetic resonance imaging (T1-weighted) in an otherwise healthy 36-year-old man with a single, nocturnal, secondarily generalized tonic-clonic seizure. The cystic lesion has not changed over 5 years and likely represents a neuroepithelial cyst.

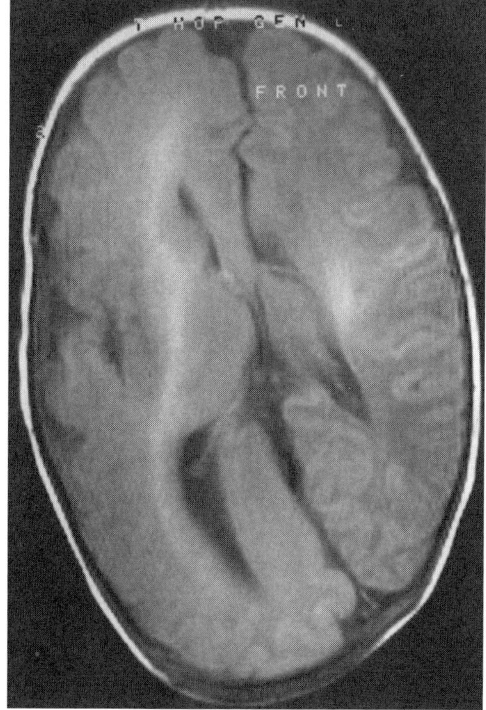

FIGURE 4.26 Magnetic resonance imaging showing right hemimegalencephaly in an 11-day-old infant having seizures.

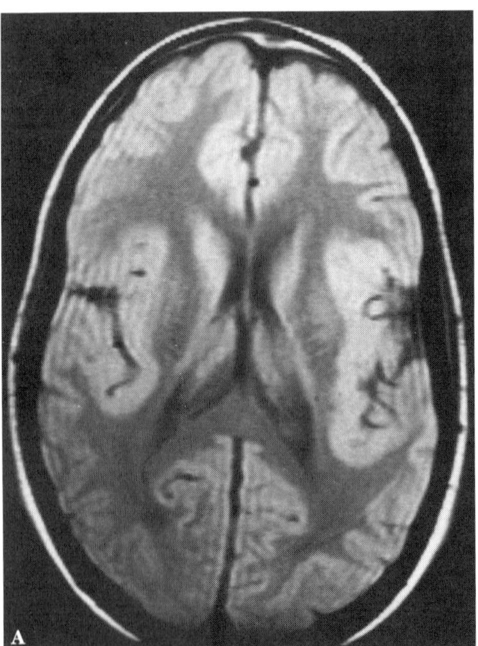

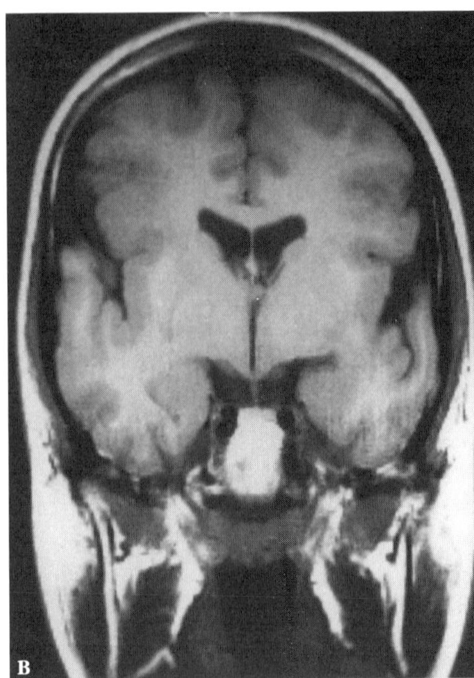

FIGURE 4.27 Axial (**A**) and coronal (**B**) magnetic resonance imaging scans in an otherwise neurologically normal 36-year-old patient having infrequent complex partial seizures. Scan shows bilateral perisylvian polymicrogyria despite the lack of muteness and lingual-buccal-facial paralysis typically seen with this disorder.

FIGURE 4.28 Axial (**A**) and sagittal (**B**) magnetic resonance imaging scans in an 11-year-old girl with seizures and headaches, showing bilateral periventricular nodular heterotopias.

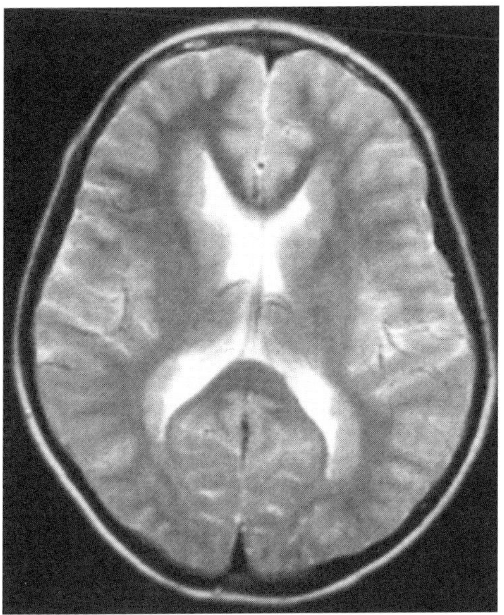

A

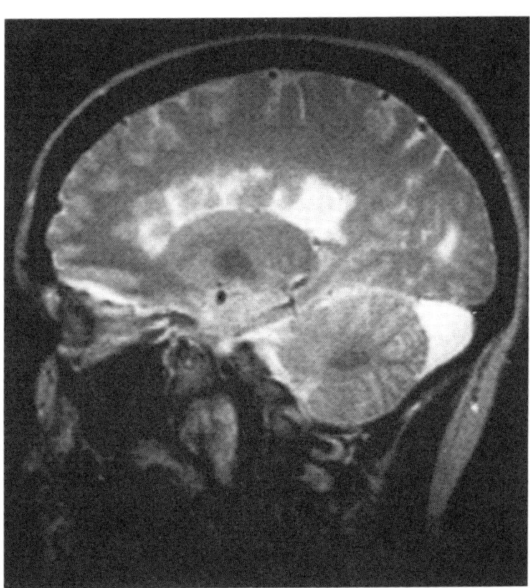

B

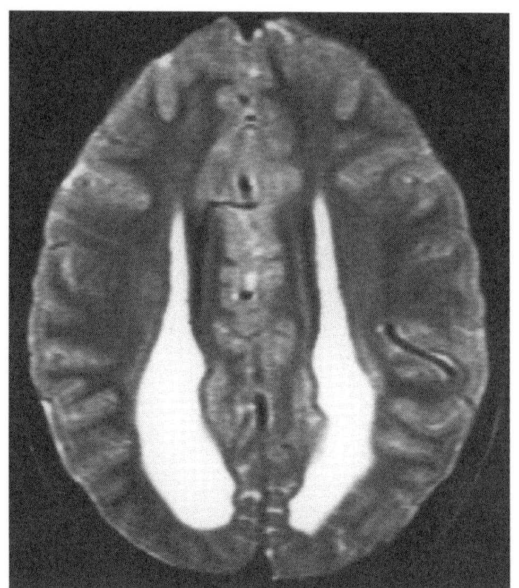

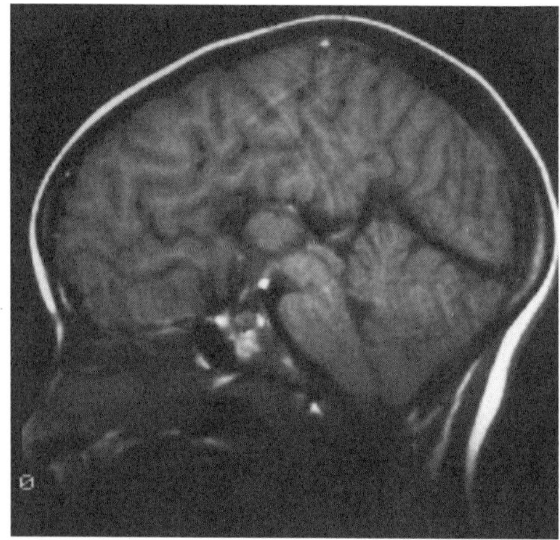

B

FIGURE 4.29 Axial (**A**) and coronal (**B**) magnetic resonance imaging scans in a 9-year-old girl with epilepsy. Scans show agenesis of the corpus callosum.

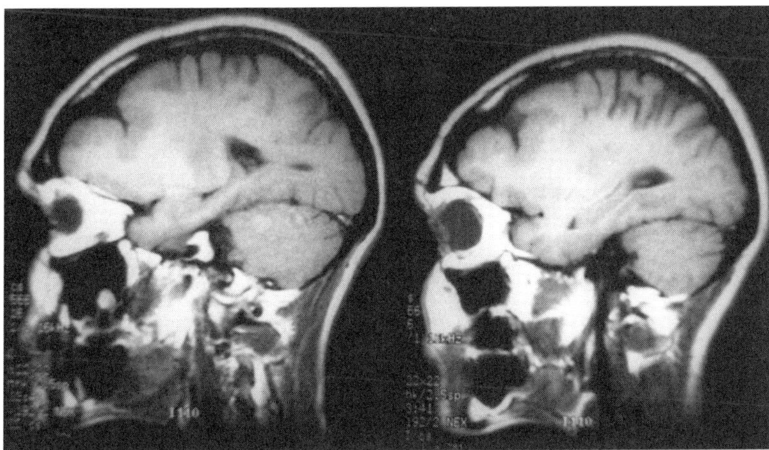

A

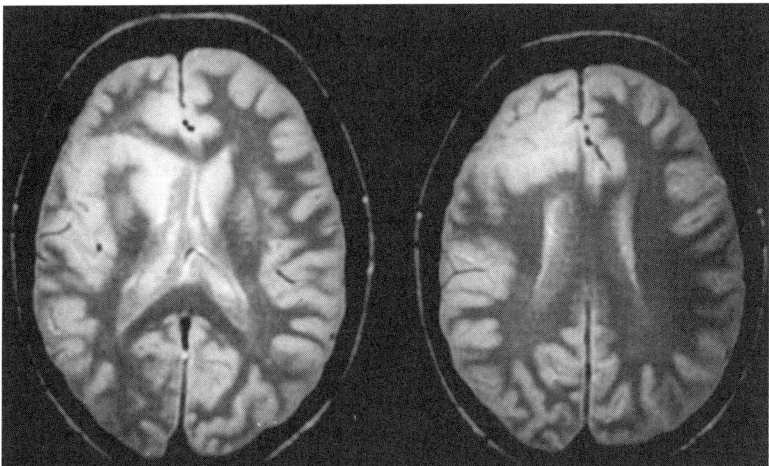

B

FIGURE 4.30 T1-weighted (**A**) and T2-weighted (**B**) magnetic resonance imaging scans showing schizencephaly and cortical dysplasia in a young woman with recent-onset complex partial seizures.

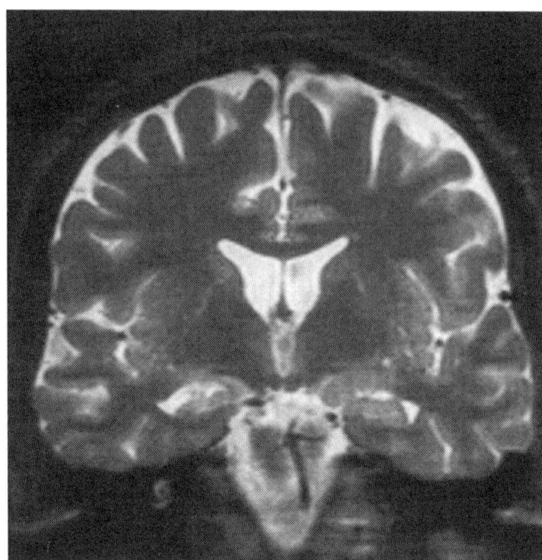

FIGURE 4.31 Coronal magnetic resonance imaging showing typical right hippocampal atrophy, disruption of internal architecture, and dilatation of temporal horn in a man with long-standing temporolimbic epilepsy due to mesial-temporal sclerosis. He had an excellent response to anterior temporal lobectomy.

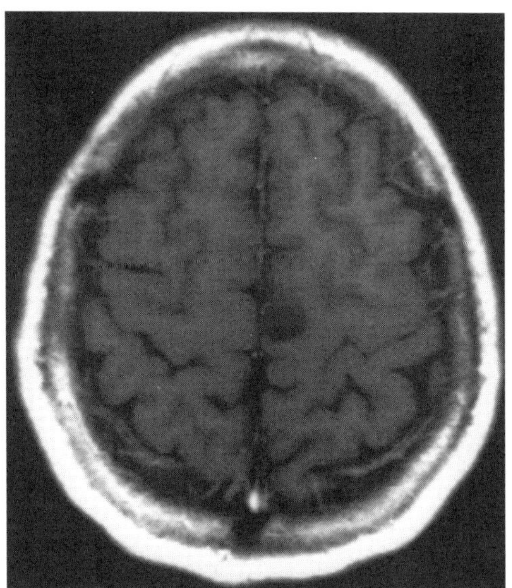

A

FIGURE 4.32 T1-weighted (**A**) and T2-weighted (**B**) magnetic resonance imaging scans in a 34-year-old man with a 10-year history of partial seizures involving shocklike sensations, elevation and abduction of the right arm with some flexion at the elbow, occasional spread to the leg, and occasional secondary generalization. At surgery, a small, superficial left parasagittal parietal lesion was found to be a ganglioglioma.

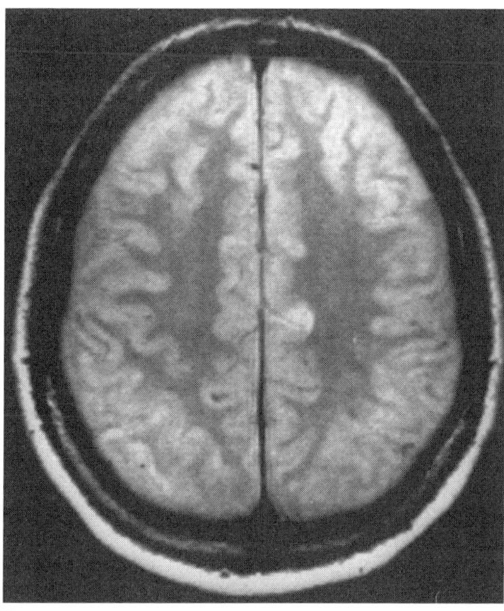

B

FIGURE 4.33 Magnetic resonance imaging showing a right mesial-temporal low-grade astrocytoma in a 29-year-old woman with recent-onset complex partial seizures. Computed tomography was normal.

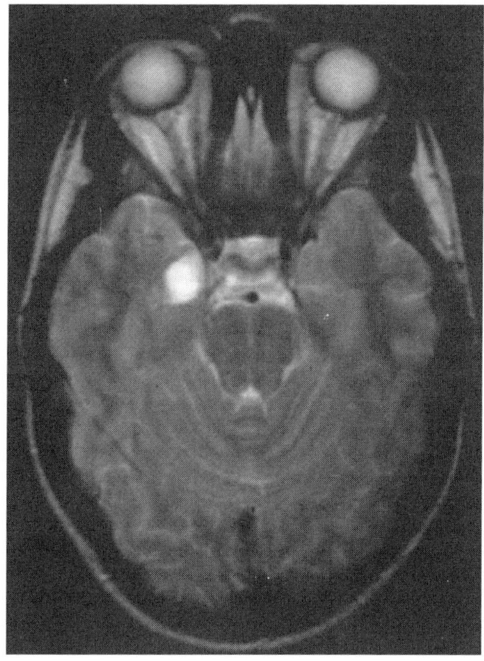

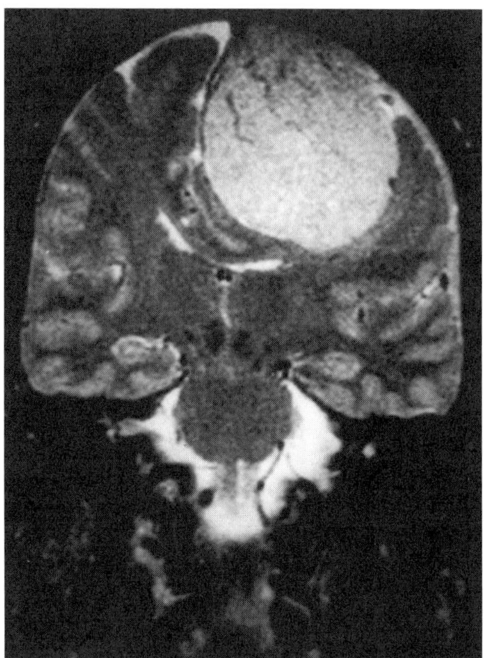

FIGURE 4.34 Magnetic resonance imaging showing massive meningioma in a 29-year-old man having his first secondarily generalized tonic-clonic seizure.

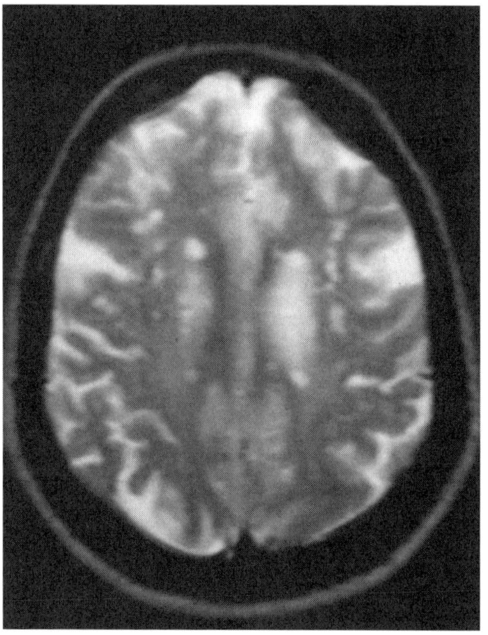

FIGURE 4.35 Magnetic resonance imaging showing multiple areas of subcortical ischemia in a 58-year-old woman with recent-onset seizures and no other obvious etiology.

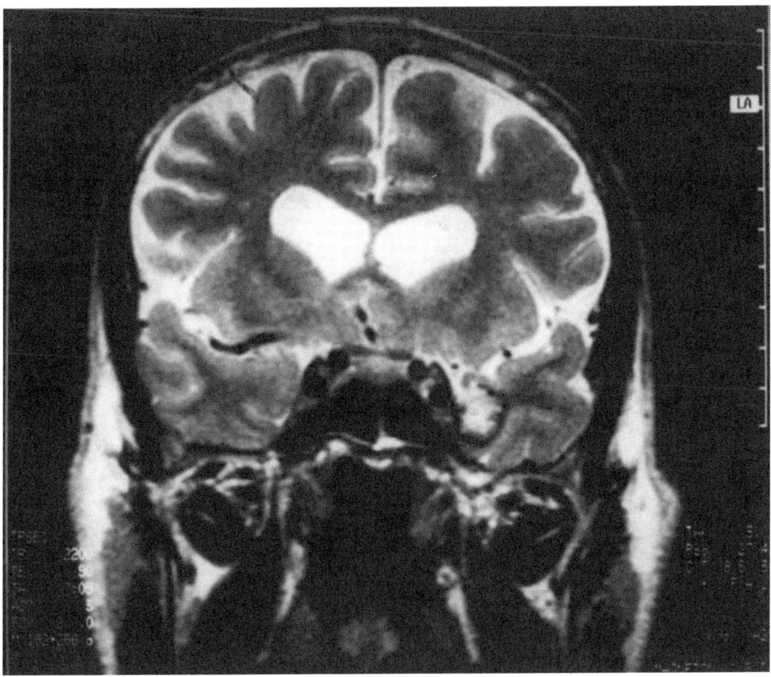

FIGURE 4.36 Coronal magnetic resonance imaging (MRI) in a 58-year-old man with a 2-year history of complex partial seizures and normal computed tomography scans. MRI shows a left temporal cavernous hemangioma.

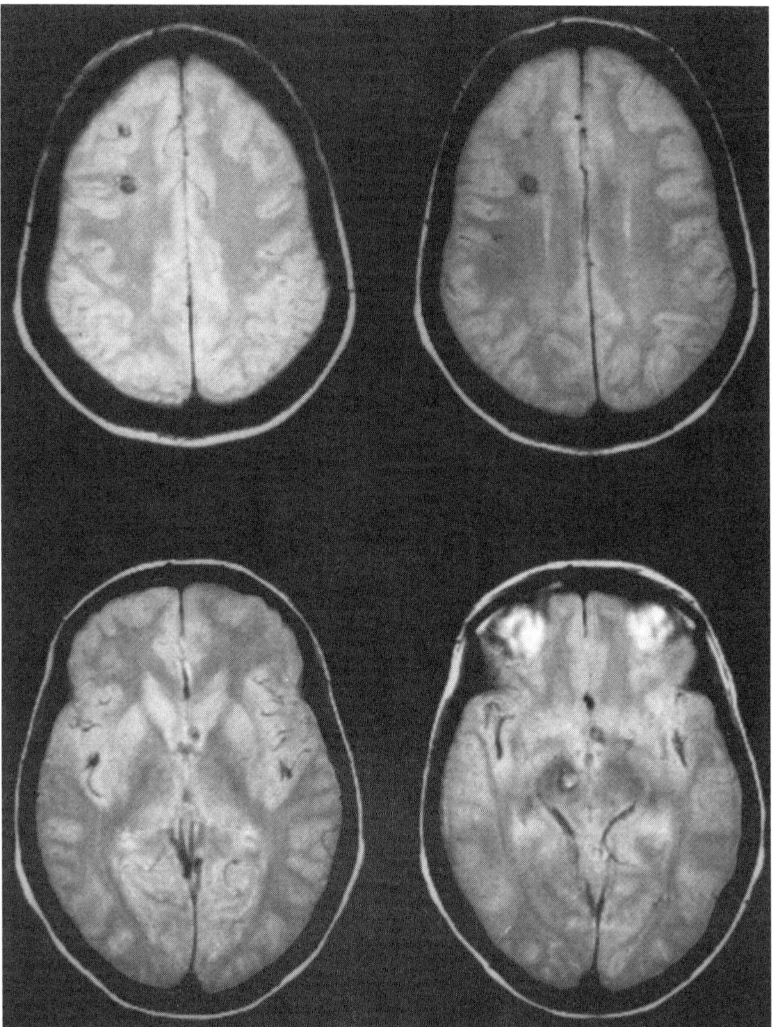

FIGURE 4.37 Magnetic resonance imaging scans showing multiple cavernous hemangiomas in a 52-year-old woman with occasional partial seizures. Computed tomography did not reveal the lesions.

Magnetic Resonance Spectroscopy

- Magnetic resonance spectroscopy provides functional or biochemical information that can be used in conjunction with structural images.
- Anatomic resolution is much less than for standard MRI.
- ^{31}P and nonwater ^{1}H spectra have been most studied.
- Phosphocreatine/inorganic phosphorous ratios decline during seizures; intracellular pH falls; adenosine triphosphate stores are only mildly depleted.
- The reduction of *N*-acetylaspartate (NAA) in seizure foci appears to correlate with neuronal loss. Increase in creatinine and choline compound peaks may reflect gliosis.
- The ratio of NAA to creatinine and choline compounds appears to decrease in the area of hippocampal sclerosis.
- The hope is that proton MRS may be more sensitive than structural MRI imaging and will be able to detect bilateral hippocampal abnormalities when side-to-side differences are minimal.
- Changes in lactate seen postictally may also be used to give dynamic information about the origin of each seizure.
- Neurotransmitters such as γ-aminobutyric acid (GABA) and glutamate can be measured.

Functional Magnetic Resonance Imaging

- fMRI is a method of visualizing discrete areas of brain activation that relies on localized increases of blood flow with increased neuronal activity, increased oxygenation of venous blood, and changes in the signal in and around blood vessels.
- When used to detect epileptic foci, fMRI has shown abnormalities in discrete brain areas during seizures and subclinical states (i.e., preictally or interictally).
- It has also been used in cognitive, speech, and motor mapping of cortical areas as part of presurgical workup.

Positron Emission Tomography

- PET is a highly specialized technique that is very expensive and available only at a small number of centers.
- It provides useful, functional, quantitative information about regional cerebral blood flow and metabolism as well as specific receptor and drug-binding data. Spatial imaging is now 3–4 mm.
- The most useful tracers are ^{18}F-2-deoxyglucose (FDG), used to measure glucose uptake, and ^{15}O-labeled water, used to measure cerebral blood flow.
- Hypometabolism on interictal FDG-PET is a sensitive way to detect temporal lobe foci even when MRI studies are negative.
- Unilateral hypometabolism on PET correlates with a good outcome after temporal lobectomy.

- Hypometabolic areas, such as in temporal neocortex and ipsilateral or contralateral cerebellum, may be found at a distance from a mesial temporal hypometabolic focus.
- Rare ictal PET scans in temporal lobe epilepsy have shown hypermetabolism in interictal hypometabolic temporal foci. The hypermetabolism may spread to subcortical areas such as the frontal and contralateral temporal lobes.
- One useful application of PET has been in children with infantile spasms, where unsuspected (usually posterior) foci have been identified, leading to successful surgical therapy.
- PET may provide insights into the pathophysiology of epilepsy and be useful for presurgical lateralization or localization of foci when MRI is negative or inconclusive. It may also be used for presurgical lateralization of language centers.

Single Photon Emission Computed Tomography

- Single photon emission computed tomography (SPECT) allows determination of cerebral blood flow in a semiquantitative fashion by measuring photons emitted from intravenously injected radiotracers (e.g., ^{99m}technetium-hexamethylpropyleneamineoxime). It is much cheaper and technically simpler than PET.
- Spatial resolution is limited to approximately 7 mm.
- One advantage of the technique is that ictal or postictal studies can be performed by injecting the tracer at the time of the seizure and scanning up to several hours later. Because the tracer remains fixed in the brain, the scan reflects cerebral blood flow at the time of tracer injection.
- The valve of SPECT in localizing temporal and extratemporal foci in surgical candidates is still uncertain.
- The tendency exists for reduced perfusion interictally, in the area of an epileptic focus, and it may extend beyond the area of the electrical focus. Certain lesions, such as gray matter heterotopias located in the white matter, have been shown to have increased perfusion interictally.
- The specificity and sensitivity of interictal SPECT is too low to make it useful for presurgical localization.
- Ictal hyperperfusion detected by SPECT provides sensitivity and specificity of 80–90% and is more promising than interictal studies.
- Ictal studies should be compared to interictal studies if possible. Postictally, there is often a period of hypoperfusion in the area of the focus before it returns to its interictal condition.
- Interpretation of the study can be difficult because several areas, presumably due to seizure spread, can show activation; the time of injection in relation to seizure onset must be known to help distinguish ictal from postictal data.
- Certain tracers have been developed to bind to specific receptors such as benzodiazepine receptors or acetylcholine receptors.

Suggested Reading

Electroencephalography and Intensive Monitoring in Epilepsy

Binnie CD, Prior PM. Electroencephalography. J Neurol Neurosurg Psychiatry 1994;57: 1308-1319.

Blume WT, Kaibara M. Atlas of Adult Electroencephalography. New York: Raven, 1994.

Drury I, Henry TR. Ictal patterns in generalized epilepsy. J Clin Neurophysiol 1993;10: 268-280.

Ebersole JS, Pacia SV. Localization of temporal lobe foci by ictal EEG patterns. Epilepsia 1996;37:386-399.

Ebner A, Hoppe M. Noninvasive electroencephalography and mesial temporal sclerosis. J Clin Neurophysiol 1995;12:23-31.

Fisch BJ. Spehlmann's EEG Primer (2nd ed). Amsterdam: Elsevier, 1991.

Foley CM, Legido A, Miles DK, et al. Diagnostic value of pediatric outpatient video-EEG. Pediatr Neurol 1995;12:120-124.

Guberman A, Couture M. Atlas of Electroencephalography. Boston: Little, Brown, 1989.

Gumnit RJ (ed). Intensive Neurodiagnostic Monitoring. Advances in Neurology. Vol 46. New York: Raven, 1987.

Klass DW, Westmoreland BF. Nonepileptogenic epileptiform electro-encephalographic activity. Ann Neurol 1985;18:627-635.

Knowlton RC, Laxer KD, Aminoff M, et al. Magnetoencephalography in partial epilepsy: clinical yield and localization accuracy. Ann Neurol 1997;42:622-631.

Lagerlund TD, Cascino GD, Cicora KM, et al. Long-term electroencephalographic monitoring for diagnosis and management of seizures. Mayo Clin Proc 1996;71:1000-1006.

Miller JW, Snyder AZ, Coben LA, et al. Clinical Electroencephalography and Related Techniques (Chapter 5). In RJ Joynt, RC Griggs (eds), Clinical Neurology. Vol. 1. Philadelphia: Lippincott-Raven, 1995; 1-115.

Mizrahi EM. Avoiding the pitfalls of EEG interpretation in childhood epilepsy. Epilepsia 1996;37(Suppl 1):S41-S51.

Newmark ME, Penry JK. Genetics of Epilepsy: A Review. New York: Raven, 1980.

Sharbrough FW. Scalp-recorded ictal patterns in focal epilepsy. J Clin Neurophysiol 1993; 10:262-267.

Sperling MR, Mendius JR, Engel J Jr. Mesial temporal spikes: a simultaneous comparison of sphenoidal, nasopharyngeal and ear electrodes. Epilepsia 1986;27:81-86.

Veldhuizen R, Binnie CD, Beintema DJ. The effect of sleep deprivation on the EEG in epilepsy. Electroencephalogr Clin Neurophysiol 1983;55:505-512.

Zivin L, Marson CA. Incidence and prognostic significance of epileptiform activity in the EEG of nonepileptic subjects. Brain 1968;91:751-778.

Neuroimaging in Epilepsy

Berkovic SF, Andermann F, Olivier A, et al. Hippocampal sclerosis in temporal lobe epilepsy demonstrated by magnetic resonance imaging. Ann Neurol 1991;29:175-182.

Cook MJ, Kilpatrick C. Imaging in epilepsy. Neurology 1994;7:123-130.

Duncan J. Positron emission tomography studies of cerebral blood flow and glucose metabolism. Epilepsia 1997;38(Suppl 10):S42-S47.

George JS, Aine CJ, Mosher JC. Mapping function in the human brain with magnetoencephalography, anatomical magnetic resonance imaging and functional magnetic resonance imaging. J Clin Neurophysiol 1995;12:406–431.

Greenberg MK, Barsan WG, Starkman S. Neuroimaging in the emergency patient presenting with seizure. Neurology 1996;47:26–32.

Hetherington H, Kuzniecky R, Pan J. Temporal lobe epilepsy at 4.1 T. Ann Neurol 1995;38: 396–404.

Jackson GD. New techniques in magnetic resonance and epilepsy. Epilepsia 1994;35(Suppl 6): 2–13.

Jackson GD, Connelly A. Magnetic resonance imaging and spectroscopy. Curr Opin Neurol 1996;9:82–88.

Kuzniecky R, de la Sayette V, Ethier R, et al. Magnetic resonance imaging in temporal lobe epilepsy: pathological correlations. Ann Neurol 1987;22:341–347.

Kuzniecky R, Hugg JW, Hetherington H, et al. Relative utility of ^{1}H spectroscopic imaging and hippocampal volumetry in the lateralization of mesial temporal lobe epilepsy. Neurology 1998;51:66–71.

Kuzniecky RI, Jackson GD. Magnetic Resonance in Epilepsy. New York: Raven, 1995.

Latchaw RE, Jack CR Jr (eds). Epilepsy: clinical evaluation, neuroimaging, surgery. Neuroimaging Clin North Am 1995;5:513–757.

Sawle GV. Imaging the head: functional imaging. J Neurol Neurosurg Psychiatry 1995; 58:132–144.

Sisodiya SM, Stevens JM, Fish DR. The demonstration of gyral abnormalities in patients with cryptogenic partial epilepsy using three-dimensional MRI. Arch Neurol 1996;53:28–34.

Theodore WH. Positron emission tomography and single photon emission computed tomography. Curr Opin Neurol 1996;9:89–92.

Van Paesschen W. Quantitative MRI of mesial temporal structures in temporal lobe epilepsy. Epilepsia 1997;38(Suppl 10):3–12.

Watson C, Jack CR Jr, Cendes F. Volumetric magnetic resonance imaging. Clinical applications and contributions to the understanding of temporal lobe epilepsy. Arch Neurol 1997;54:1521–1531.

5 Principles of Pharmacotherapy

Pharmacokinetic Principles

Terms

Important definitions that should be understood include the following:

- *Pharmacokinetics*: The quantitative aspects of drug absorption, distribution, and elimination. An understanding of these processes is important in the optimal use of AEDs and in the understanding of the factors that influence drug plasma concentrations.
- *Area under the curve* (AUC): A reflection of the course of plasma concentration over time; reflects the interplay between administered dose, rate of absorption, distribution, and metabolism (or renal excretion) (Figure 5.1).
- *Tmax*: Time of maximal plasma concentration after administration.
- *Cmax*: Peak concentration after a single dose.
- *Biological half-life* ($T_{1/2}$): The time taken for the plasma concentration of a drug to decrease by 50% is $T_{1/2} = 0.693\,V_d/\text{clearance}$. This relationship shows that the half-life is inversely related to the clearance, and the larger the volume of distribution (V_d), the longer the half-life. The effective half-life of a drug may not be proportional to the biological half-life (e.g., with vigabatrin).
- *Steady state*: A condition when absorption and elimination are in equilibrium and the mean drug concentration is constant from one dose interval to the next. Generally, steady-state conditions are achieved after five to six half-lives have lapsed. It takes five to six half-lives for a drug to be eliminated from the body when dosing is stopped and five to six half-lives to reach a new steady state when the daily dose is changed.
- *Drug clearance*: The total removal of a drug per unit of time; may involve renal or hepatic clearance, or both (Table 5.1).

Absorption

- Most AEDs are well absorbed by passive transport in the intestinal tract. The lipid solubility of drugs and the time of contact with the absorptive surface determine the amount of drug absorbed. Although administration with food

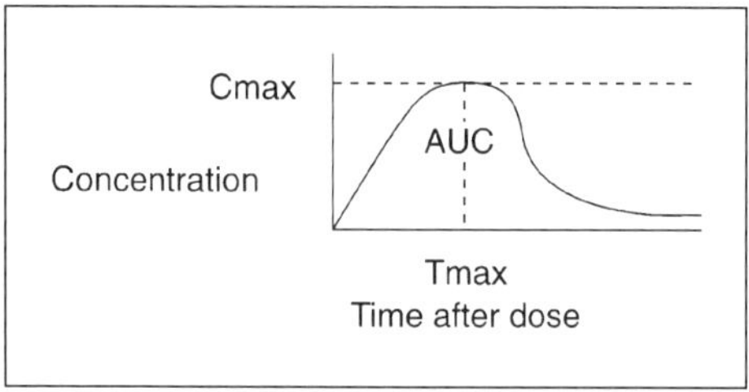

FIGURE 5.1 Relationship between plasma concentration of an antiepileptic drug and time after oral administration. (Cmax = peak plasma concentration of the drug following a single dose; AUC = area under the curve; Tmax = time interval between administration of the dose and achievement of maximum plasma concentration.)

does not impair the extent of absorption of AEDs, it may delay the time of absorption. This delay is not clinically significant.

- Absorption occurs predominantly in the gut.
- Sustained-release forms reduce the peak-trough fluctuations and may allow less frequent dosing.
- Rectal administration of diazepam or valproate can achieve therapeutic levels.
- Drug interactions at the absorption level generally are not significant; however, the administration of phenytoin with antacids may retard its absorption, and tube feedings may reduce phenytoin absorption.

TABLE 5.1 Approximate Time to Achieve Steady State

Drug	*Steady-State Time (Days)*
Phenytoin	7-20
Carbamazepine	3-5
Phenobarbital	10-30
Primidone	2-5
Valproate	2-5*
Ethosuximide	7-12
Clobazam	4-5
Gabapentin	2-5
Vigabatrin	2-5*
Lamotrigine	3-10
Topiramate	3-6
Tiagabine	1-2

*Once- to twice-a-day dosing is possible despite short half-life because the effective half-life is longer than the biological half-life.

Distribution

- The volume of distribution of an antiepileptic drug depends on its water and lipid solubility, binding to plasma proteins, drug interactions, and the amount of body fat in the person taking the drug.
- The lipid solubility of a drug determines its transport across biological membranes. Transport is by passive diffusion along concentration gradients, but active transport mechanisms may also play a role.
- The volume of distribution of a drug is one of the factors that influence plasma concentration and half-life of a drug.
- Highly protein-bound drugs include phenytoin, valproate, benzodiazepines, carbamazepine, and tiagabine.

Clearance

- Most AEDs (phenytoin, carbamazepine, primidone, valproate, ethosuximide, the benzodiazepines, and lamotrigine) are eliminated by hepatic metabolism.
- Phenobarbital, felbamate, topiramate, and tiagabine are partially eliminated by hepatic metabolism.
- The main types of enzymatic reactions include oxidation, reduction, and hydrolysis (phase I reactions). Most of the AEDs are metabolized by oxidative reactions, through the cytochrome P450 enzyme system, to less active metabolites. Conjugation (phase II) reactions, usually with glucuronic acid, subsequently result in more polar inert metabolites, which are more easily excreted by the kidney. Most antiepileptic drug interactions (pharmacokinetic) occur at the level of hepatic metabolism.
- Protein-binding changes and concurrent administration of hepatic enzyme inducers or inhibitors influence drug metabolism and plasma concentration.
- AEDs are generally eliminated (cleared) by first-order kinetics, with a linear relationship between the dose of the administered drug and the plasma concentration. Phenytoin clearance is by zero-order (saturation, Michaelis-Menten) kinetics, implying that its elimination is dose-dependent. To prevent disproportionate increases in the plasma concentration of phenytoin with increasing doses, dose increases by 30- to 50-mg increments are more appropriate than increases by larger amounts.
- Valproate protein binding decreases with higher concentrations. The relative clearance increases with higher doses, because clearance is dependent on the free fraction of drug.
- Gabapentin and vigabatrin are excreted unchanged by the kidney.

Pharmacokinetic Interactions

Drug interactions that result in altered concentration of a drug, as a result of interaction at the absorption site or with its binding or elimination, are known as *pharmacokinetic interactions*. Most are due to induction or inhibition of the enzymatic biotransformation of the drugs. AED interactions are more common with the drugs that are eliminated by hepatic metabolism. Interactions may also occur between AEDs and drugs used for other medical conditions.

Pharmacodynamic Interactions

Pharmacodynamic interactions are drug interactions that occur at receptor sites and are not related to changes in the amount of drug delivered. This type of interaction may have an additive, synergistic, or antagonistic effect. Some neurotoxic interactions of the AEDs are pharmacodynamic and are more difficult to quantify than kinetic interactions.

Measurement of Plasma Concentration

- In treating the patient with epilepsy, clinical response and lack of unacceptable side effects are more useful indications of the optimal dose of an antiepileptic drug than is the plasma concentration. This is particularly true for new drugs, such as vigabatrin, gabapentin, lamotrigine, topiramate, felbamate, and tiagabine, whose therapeutic levels have not been well-defined. Therapeutic drug levels are not based on scientific data but on clinical experience. The ideal "therapeutic" level varies from patient to patient and possibly for different seizure types.
- When the drug level is assessed, one must also determine whether it may represent a peak or trough level based on the time of sampling in relation to the dosing interval. Plasma levels are often measured under the following conditions:
  - After initiation of therapy, to assess steady-state level
  - After change in drug dose once a new steady state is achieved
  - When compliance should be checked
  - When kinetic drug interactions are suspected
  - In the presence of intercurrent illnesses that may alter the bioavailability or elimination of the drug, such as renal disease, hepatic disease, or malabsorption
  - During pregnancy, because changes in protein binding and metabolism may result in lower plasma concentrations that may require dose adjustment
  - If the patient develops subtle symptoms that may be related to drug toxicity
  - During AED clinical research trials
- When interpreting blood level data, the following factors that may influence the level should be considered:
  - Age of the patient
  - Genetic variability in drug metabolism
  - Individualized therapeutic window
  - Drug interactions
  - Presence of disease states
  - Pregnancy
  - Compliance
  - Environmental factors (e.g., smoking may induce cytochrome P450 system)
- Plasma level measurements generally measure total drug concentration (free + protein-bound drug), but only the unbound or free drug is pharmacologi-

cally active. This is particularly important for highly protein-bound drugs, such as phenytoin or valproate, with which protein-binding interactions may occur. In addition, hepatic or renal disease or other hypoalbuminemic states may increase the relative free fraction of these drugs, and the total drug concentration may underestimate the pharmacologically active portion. In these situations, measuring free plasma concentrations is worthwhile.

- Knowledge of the mechanisms of action of AEDs is important for predicting possible side effects and for choosing rational drug combinations (see next section). The mechanisms are shown in Table 5.2.

Preclinical Evaluation of Antiepileptic Drugs

- No single laboratory test or animal model accurately predicts the efficacy and toxicity of a chemical compound in humans. One cannot predict the efficacy of an AED based solely on its mechanism(s) of action. Unidentified mechanisms may play a role.
- Testing of potential AEDs can be performed in seizure-prone animals (e.g., mice with audiogenic seizures, tottering mice, E1 mouse, or photosensitive baboon Papio papio) or can be performed after injection of a known convulsant into an animal.

TABLE 5.2 Antiepileptic Drugs: Main Mechanisms of Action

	Sodium Channel Blockade/ Modulation	*Calcium Channel Blockade/ Modulation*	*GABA Enhancement*	*Glutamate Receptor Blockade/ Modulation*
Phenytoin	+	-	-	-
Carbamazepine	+	-	-	-
Phenobarbital	+	-	+	-
Primidone	+	-	+	-
Valproic acid	+	-	+	-
Ethosuximide	-	+	-	-
Benzodiazepines (e.g., clobazam)	+	-	+	-
Vigabatrin	-	-	+	-
Gabapentin	-	-	+	-
Lamotrigine	+	+	-	-
Topiramate	+	-	+	+ (AMPA)
Tiagabine	-	-	+	-
Felbamate	±	-	+	+ (NMDA)

AMPA = aminomethylisoxazole propionate; GABA = γ-aminobutyric acid; NMDA = *N*-methyl-D-aspartate.

- Acute toxicity is usually established in mice or rats by assessing performance on a number of tests, including the Rotorod test, gait and stance tests, and muscle tone tests, and by determining the median toxic dose (TD_{50}).
- The pentylenetetrazol (PTZ) model has been used to screen compounds for their effect on seizure thresholds. Absence of a clonic seizure after a subcutaneous injection of PTZ is an indication that the seizure threshold can be raised. Compounds effective in this model may offer protection against clinical absence seizures. Carbamazepine and phenytoin have little effect. Ethosuximide and valproate have a protective effect. The median effective dose (ED_{50}) can be established for each compound.
- In the maximal electroshock test, abolition of the hind limb tonic extensor component of the electrically induced seizure is indicative of protection against seizure spread. Compounds effective in this model may offer protection against tonic-clonic and partial seizures. Carbamazepine and phenytoin are active in this model.
- The kindling model of epilepsy may be useful in the identification of compounds that may be effective against complex partial seizures and tonic-clonic seizures.
- Drugs useful in the treatment of myoclonic seizures (e.g., valproate and the benzodiazepines) are effective in the PTZ model.
- The hippocampal slice model can be used to study the effect of chemical compounds on bursting behavior of hippocampal neurones. Bursting can be reduced or abolished by the benzodiazepines, phenytoin, carbamazepine, valproate, and the barbiturates.
- The major mechanisms of action(s) that have been identified for the various AEDs (see Table 5.2) include
  - Modulation of voltage-gated sodium channels
  - Modulation of calcium channels
  - Enhancement of GABA-mediated inhibition
  - Inhibition of the effect of excitatory amino acids on *N*-methyl-D-aspartate (NMDA) and aminomethylisoxazole propionate (AMPA) receptors

Principles of Epilepsy Treatment and Drug Selection

Goals of treatment that should be kept in mind and explained to the patient are

- Complete control of seizures
- Minimal side effects from AEDs
- Optimal quality of life

Initiating Treatment

- Some patients who have seizures only every few years, occasional nocturnal seizures, benign syndromes such as benign rolandic epilepsy of childhood, or nondisabling brief simple partial seizures may not require treatment.

- The drug factors to be considered when choosing an AED are
  - Efficacy
  - Side effects (idiosyncratic/allergic; acute dose-related; chronic effects on tissues, organs, and cognitive function; teratogenicity)
  - Ease of use (e.g., dosing, interactions, pharmacokinetics, and need for serum levels)
  - Cost
- Therapy must be *individualized*, taking into account the following factors:
  - Importance to the patient of having *complete* seizure control.
  - Susceptibility of the patient to specific side effects (partially based on side effects with previous AEDs). For example, valproic acid is best avoided in obese individuals; phenytoin is not a good choice in young women due to cosmetic side effects.
  - Presence of other illnesses.
  - Patient's neurologic status.
  - Likelihood of the patient being compliant (single or double daily doses are best in noncompliant individuals).
  - Affordability.
- When initiating treatment, explain to the patient that
  - Treatment is not curative; it only suppresses seizures.
  - The first drug might not stop seizures, and dosage adjustments or a change to another drug may be required.
  - An interval of at least five times the average interval between seizures will be necessary to judge the efficacy of the drug.
  - Patients must renew their drugs in good time, must not permit generic substitution without their doctor's knowledge, and must investigate any potential drug interactions for other required medications, even with over-the-counter medications such as cold remedies.
- Emphasize the importance of the following patient-dependent factors in seizure control: avoiding sleep deprivation; avoiding undue stress; avoiding overuse of alcohol or recreational drugs such as cocaine, which can provoke seizures; good compliance.
- The authors' current drugs of choice and properties of the main AEDs are shown in Tables 5.3 and 5.4.
- Treatment is begun with *monotherapy*. The advantages of monotherapy are
  - Fewer side effects
  - No drug interactions
  - Reduced cost of medication
  - Reduced teratogenic effects
  - Better compliance
  - Improved quality of life
- In patients with more than one seizure type (especially if absences, atonic seizures, or myoclonic seizures are included), a broad-spectrum drug such as

TABLE 5.3 Antiepileptic Drugs of Choice

Seizure Type	*First Choice Monotherapy*	*Other Drugs with Efficacy for Seizure Type*
Generalized		
Tonic-clonic	VPA, CBZ, PHT	CLB,* GBP, LTG, PB, PRM, TGB, TPM, VGB*
Absence	VPA, ESM	AZM, CLB, FBM, LTG, TPM
Myoclonic	VPA	AZM, CLB, CZP, FBM, LTG, TPM, ketogenic diet (pediatric), steroids (pediatric infantile spasms)
Atonic	VPA	CLB, FBM, LTG, TPM, ketogenic diet (pediatric)
Partial		
Simple or complex ± secondary generalization	CBZ, PHT	CLB, GBP, LTG, PB, PRM, TGB, TPM, VGB, VPA
Syndromes		
Benign rolandic epilepsy	CBZ	CLB, GBP, PHT
Juvenile myoclonic epilepsy	VPA	CLB, LTG, TPM, CBZ or PHT (for generalized tonic-clonic seizures)
Lennox-Gastaut	VPA	CLB, CZP, FBM, LTG, TPM, VGB, ketogenic diet (pediatric)
West syndrome (infantile spasms)	VGB, ACTH	CLB, CZP, LTG, steroids, VPA

ACTH = adrenocorticotropic hormone; AZM = acetazolamide; CBZ = carbamazepine; CLB = clobazam; CZP = clonazepam; ESM = ethosuximide; FBM = felbamate; GBP = gabapentin; LTG = lamotrigine; PB = phenobarbital; PHT = phenytoin; PRM = primidone; TGB = tiagabine; TPM = topiramate; VGB = vigabatrin; VPA = valproic acid.
*Not marketed in the United States.

valproic acid, clobazam, lamotrigine, or possibly topiramate is an appropriate first choice.

- Expect certain epileptic syndromes, such as temporal lobe epilepsy due to mesial-temporal sclerosis, West syndrome, severe myoclonic epilepsy of infancy, and Lennox-Gastaut syndrome, to be difficult to control.
- Polytherapy controls seizures for only about 10% of patients for whom two first-line AEDs have been unsuccessful as monotherapy.
- Normally, two first-line agents are used in monotherapy before consideration of adding a second drug. When adding a second or third drug to a regimen, the concept of *rational polytherapy* is recommended, even though there is

TABLE 5.4 Principal Antiepileptic Drugs

Drug	*Average Adult Dose (mg/day)*	*Therapeutic Serum Levels μmol/liter (μg/ml)*	*$T_{1/2}$ (hrs)*	*Protein Binding (%)*	*Main Side Effects*
Phenytoin (Dilantin)	350	40–80 (10–20)	24 ± 12	75–95	Ataxia, blurred vision, gingival hyperplasia, hirsutism, sedation
Carbamazepine (Tegretol, Tegretol-XR, Tegretol CR, Carbatrol)	1,000	20–50 (4–12)	5–12	75–80	Ataxia, diplopia, hepatic, blood dyscrasia
Phenobarbital	120	80–200 (20–40)	25–150	50	Sedation, cognitive impairment
Primidone (Mysoline)	750	15–40 (3–8); 80–200 (20–40) as phenobarbital	10–25	0–50	Sedation, cognitive impairment
Valproic acid/divalproex sodium (Depakene, Depakote, Epival)	1,500	350–700 (50–100)	12 ± 6	90	Severe hepatic toxicity, tremor, gastrointestinal upset, weight gain, hair loss
Ethosuximide (Zarontin)	1,000	350–700 (40–100)	40–60 in adults; 30–40 in children	0	Sedation, blood dyscrasia
Clonazepam (Klonopin, Rivotril)	2–6	0.005–0.070 μg/ml	20–70	85	Sedation

TABLE 5.4 *Continued*

Drug	*Average Adult Dose (mg/day)*	*Therapeutic Serum Levels μmol/liter (μg/ml)*	$T_{1/2}$ *(hrs)*	*Protein Binding (%)*	*Main Side Effects*
Clobazam* (Frisium)	20–40	Clobazam: 0.5–1.0; *N*-desmethyl clobazam: 5–10	Clobazam: 18; *N*-desmethyl clobazam: 42	85	Sedation, ataxia
Vigabatrin* (Sabril)	2–4 g/day	—	5–8 (GABA-T takes 3–5 days to be resynthesized)	0	Dizziness, depression, psychosis (2–4%), weight gain, retinal degeneration with long-term use (in possibly 20%)
Lamotrigine (Lamictal)	100–200 (concurrent valproate); 300–400 (monotherapy or valproate + inducer); 500–600 (combined with inducer)	—	48–60 with VPA; 24–30 with monotherapy; 15 with hepatic enzyme inducers	55	Skin rash (severe in ~1:100 children and 1:300 adults), ataxia, dizziness, headache, insomnia
Gabapentin (Neurontin)	1,800–3,600	—	5–8	0	Fatigue, drowsiness, dizziness, ataxia
Topiramate (Topamax)	200–400	—	12–24	15	Cognitive impairment, weight loss, kidney stones (1.5%)

Tiagabine (Gabitril)	32–56	—	4–8; 2–3 with hepatic enzyme inducers	95	Headache, drowsiness, fatigue
Felbamate (Felbatol)	2,400	—	13–23	25	Severe, potentially fatal hepatotoxicity or aplastic anemia; weight loss, insomnia

GABA = γ-aminobutyric acid; $T_{1/2}$ = biological half-life; VPA = valproic acid.
*Not released in the United States.

no hard evidence for its use. Rational polytherapy implies that drugs with different mechanisms of action, such as carbamazepine and vigabatrin (or clobazam or gabapentin), are best combined (see Table 5.2). Other features of rational polytherapy are taking advantage of pharmacokinetic properties (e.g., elevation of *N*-desmethyl clobazam levels by carbamazepine or elevation of carbamazepine 10,11-epoxide levels by valproate) or offsetting side effects (e.g., weight gain on valproate and weight loss on topiramate).

- Dose is increased very gradually to reach the lowest recommended maintenance dose, unless a quick response is necessary. Phenytoin and gabapentin are the drugs that can be titrated most rapidly.
- Steady state is reached at five half-lives after the last dosage increment; only after reaching steady state can efficacy be judged.
- Pharmacokinetic principles (see preceding section) should be taken into account when prescribing AEDs. During a 24-hour dosing interval, peak and trough concentrations occur according to the dosing interval. Normally, drugs are prescribed every half-life or every half half-life. AEDs with relatively long half-lives that can be given once daily are phenytoin, phenobarbital, clobazam, clonazepam, vigabatrin (effective half-life is not dependent on elimination half-life), lamotrigine in monotherapy or combined with valproate, and possibly topiramate.
- Other pharmacokinetic factors that may influence dosing with individual drugs include the following:
  - Autoinduction of carbamazepine, which occurs 4–6 weeks after initiation of therapy and may require a dose increase
  - Shift from first-order to zero-order kinetics with phenytoin, which requires dosage increments of 30–50 mg in higher daily dose ranges
  - Saturable gastrointestinal absorption of gabapentin, which limits absorption at doses above 3,000 mg per day
  - Diminished protein binding of valproic acid at higher blood levels, which increases the free fraction of the drug
  - Active metabolites of primidone, carbamazepine, and clobazam, whose concentrations increase in combination with inducing agents
  - Renal excretion of gabapentin and vigabatrin, which requires dosage adjustments for creatinine clearance changes (e.g., in older patients or in patients with renal failure)
- Be aware of drug interactions among AEDs and between AEDs and other drugs (Tables 5.5 and 5.6).

Monitoring

- Pretreatment platelets, blood urea nitrogen (BUN), creatinine, and complete blood cell counts (CBCs) should be taken, and liver function should be tested; all should be remeasured at approximately 3 months and after 1 year. Serum folate, CBC, calcium, and alkaline phosphatase should be checked occasionally in patients taking phenytoin. Routine monitoring of CBC and liver function tests has not been of use in predicting serious hepatic or hematologic

TABLE 5.5 Drug Interactions Affecting Antiepileptic Drugs

Added Drug	*Levels of Antiepileptic Drug Affected*								
	PHT	*CBZ*	*VPA*	*PB*	*CLB*	*LTG*	*TGB*	*TPM*	*FBM*
PHT	—	↓ CBZ; ↑ 10,11-epoxide	Total ↓; free ↑	↓ or no change	Rarely ↑	↓	↓	↓	↓
CBZ	↑ or ↓	↓	↓	↑ or ↓	N-D-CLB ↑	↓	↓	↓	↓
VPA	Total ↓; free ↑	↑ 10,11-epoxide	—	↑	—	↑	—	—	↑
PB	↑ or ↓	↓ CBZ; ↑ 10,11-epoxide	↓	—	—	↓	↓	↓	—
CLB	Rarely ↑	—	Rarely ↑	—	—	—	—	—	—
VGB	20% ↓	—	—	—	—	—	—	—	—
FBM	↑	↓ CBZ; ↑ 10,11-epoxide	↑	—	—	—	—	—	—
Verapamil	↑	↑	—	—	—	—	—	—	—
Diltiazem	↑	↑	—	—	—	—	—	—	—
Erythromycin; clarithromycin	—	↑	—	—	—	—	—	—	—
Ciprofloxacin	↓	—	—	—	—	—	—	—	—
INH	↑	↑	↑	—	—	—	—	—	—
Ticlopidine	↑	—	—	—	—	—	—	—	—
Fluoxetine	↑	↑	—	—	—	—	—	—	—
Cimetidine	↑	↑	—	—	—	—	—	—	—
Dexamethasone	↓	—	—	—	—	—	—	—	—
Rifampin	↓	—	—	—	—	—	—	—	—
Antacids	↓	—	—	—	—	—	—	—	—
ASA	Free ↑	—	—	—	—	—	—	—	—

ASA = acetyl salicylic acid; CBZ = carbamazepine; CLB = clobazam; FBM = felbamate; INH = isoniazid; LTG = lamotrigine; N-D CLB = *N*-desmethyl clobazam; PHT = phenytoin; PB = phenobarbital; PRIM = primidone; TGB = tiagabine; TPM = topiramate; VPA = valproic acid; VGB = vigabatrin.

TABLE 5.6 Drug Interactions: Effects of Antiepileptic Drugs on Other Drugs

Drug Affected	*Antiepileptic Added*			
	Phenytoin	*Carbamazepine*	*Phenobarbital*	*Valproic Acid*
Benzodiazepines		↓ Pharmacologic effects	—	↑ Levels
Clozapine	↓	↓	—	Slightly ↑
Cyclosporine	↓	↓	—	—
Dexamethasone	↓	—	↓	—
Digoxin	↓	—	—	—
Doxycycline	↓	↓	—	—
Felodipine	↓	↓	—	—
Furosemide	↓ Effect	—	↓ Effect	—
Haloperidol	↓	↓	—	—
Lithium	—	↑ Toxicity	—	—
Oral contraceptives	↓	↓	↓	—
Phenothiazines	↓	—	↓	↑
Theophylline	↓	↓	—	—
Tricyclic antidepressants	—	↓	—	Possibly ↑
Protease inhibitors (e.g., saquinavir)	↓	↓	↓	—
Warfarin	↓	↓	↓	—

toxicity. However, routine monitoring may be valuable in patients on valproate, at high risk for hepatotoxicity (younger than 2 years old, on polytherapy), or in patients on felbamate.

- Serum AED levels (Table 5.7) should be measured for the traditional drugs after steady state is reached and the patient appears to be well controlled. Morning predose trough levels or late afternoon trough levels should be used when assessing efficacy, and peak levels should be used when assessing dose-related toxicity. Routine measurement may be considered periodically (every year or two) to assess compliance, even if patients are fully controlled. The routine levels obtained are total levels (bound and free) (Table 5.8).
- Levels of valproate tend to fluctuate more and correlate less with therapeutic response than most other traditional AEDs.

TABLE 5.7 Indications for Obtaining Serum Antiepileptic Drug Levels

At initiation of therapy (steady state) to set a baseline when patient is well controlled
To determine compliance
To determine dose-related toxicity (peak levels), especially when patients are on multiple drugs
To diagnose dose-related toxicity in patients who cannot communicate their symptoms (e.g., young children or the mentally handicapped)
To determine the effects of drug interactions when drugs that potentially interact are added or discontinued
In all uncontrolled patients
In special situations where free or total levels may change, such as hypoalbuminemia, pregnancy, uremia, hepatic failure, gastrointestinal illness—especially if seizure control decreases

- In instances of suspected dose-related toxicity with carbamazepine, 10,11-epoxide levels should be measured if carbamazepine levels are not elevated.
- Levels of clobazam and its *N*-desmethyl metabolite are rarely useful, since a therapeutic range has not been defined. However, *N*-desmethyl levels higher than 10 μmol/liter usually correlate with dose-related toxicity.
- The therapeutic range for an AED is only a guideline; it differs somewhat for individual patients and perhaps for different seizure types.
- If the patient is well controlled but levels are "subtherapeutic," it is not essential to increase the dose unless it is extremely important for that individual to have maximal assurance of remaining seizure-free.
- If patients have levels above the usual therapeutic range and do not appear to have adverse effects, dose does not have to be reduced. However, subtle cog-

TABLE 5.8 Situations in which Free Antiepileptic Drug (AED) Levels May Be Useful

Hypoalbuminemia
Older patients
Pregnancy
Uremia
Concurrent drugs that may involve displacement of AEDs from protein binding (e.g., salicylates, valproate)

Note: It is worth measuring free levels only with highly bound AEDs, such as phenytoin and valproate.

nitive side effects should be looked for in such patients, and family members should be questioned in this regard.
- Considerations if AED blood levels are subtherapeutic:
  - Inadequate dose
  - Noncompliance
  - Excessive peak-trough variation
  - Genetically fast metabolism
  - Induction of hepatic enzymes (e.g., by other AEDs, alcohol)
  - Poor absorption (e.g., concurrent antacids, gastrointestinal disease)

Long-Term Follow-Up

- Noncompliance is frequently seen in epilepsy patients. It increases with polytherapy, when patients have side effects from their drugs, in teenagers, and in patients with memory deficits.
- Substitution of *generic preparations* of AEDs may lead to escape from control or AED toxicity due to differences in bioavailability between generic and brand name formulations and among different batches of generic drugs. When feasible, brand name preparations, which are more tightly controlled, should be used. Generic substitution is more likely to lead to problems in patients with difficult to control or brittle seizures, drugs with a narrow therapeutic range, poorly water-soluble drugs, and drugs with nonlinear kinetics (e.g., phenytoin).
- Rarely used adjuvant drugs may be useful in certain circumstances. For example, flunarizine (Sibelium), which is not released in the United States, has antiepileptic properties and may be useful in the epileptic patient with migraine. Clorazepate dipotassium (Tranxene) is a tranquilizer with some antiepileptic activity. Piracetam in large doses has been found to be useful in cortical myoclonus following anoxic encephalopathy or in some cases of progressive myoclonus epilepsy. Diarrhea is a side effect. Piracetam is not marketed in North America.

Ketogenic Diet

- The *ketogenic* diet has been used successfully in some resistant pediatric cases for more than 70 years but involves severe carbohydrate restriction, is difficult to enforce, and is unpalatable and unhealthy due to its high fat content.
- The diet may work by favorably influencing cerebral energy supply and thereby raising seizure threshold or by inducing acidosis. The mechanism of action is unknown.
- Three diets have been used: the classic ketogenic diet, medium-chain triglycerides, and modified medium-chain triglyceride diet.
- It is used mainly for children with epileptic encephalopathies, such as Lennox-Gastaut syndrome, with intractable mixed seizures. It may work for a variety of seizure types.
- About one-third to two-thirds of patients derive benefit, at times dramatic, when the diet is used in addition to their AEDs.

- Patients who respond may be able to have their AEDs discontinued.
- Mood and activity level may improve.
- Extensive parent training and child monitoring are necessary.
- Potential side effects include reduced bone mass, renal stones, hypoproteinemia, hyperlipidemia, hair loss, metabolic encephalopathy, behavioral disturbances, hemolytic anemia, hyperuricemia, and refusal to eat. A study of 52 children treated with the classic ketogenic diet found a 10% incidence of serious side effects.
- It should be used with caution in children on valproic acid, due to potential renal tubular acidosis and hepatotoxicity; carnitine supplementation should be considered.

Intractability

- Intractability is a loosely defined concept that takes into account seizure frequency, seizure severity (e.g., impaired consciousness, injury, prolonged postictal dysfunction), and the psychosocial consequences of epilepsy and its drug treatment. Patients whose seizures are frequent enough or severe enough to cause significant negative effects on quality of life despite treatment with at least two appropriate AEDs in adequate doses for a period of time to judge efficacy may be considered intractable.
- In intractable patients, consider the following potential causes:
    - Wrong diagnosis (e.g., syncope or pseudoseizures rather than epilepsy)
    - Pseudoseizures in addition to true seizures
    - Inadequate AED levels due to one of the causes mentioned above (including intermittent noncompliance, which may not be evident at the time blood samples are taken)
    - Inattention to lifestyle factors such as sleep deprivation and alcohol, which could provoke seizures
    - Underlying progressive brain lesion or metabolic disorder (e.g., tumor, mitochondrial encephalomyelopathy)
    - Intrinsically intractable epileptic syndrome (see Table 2.1)
    - Antiepileptic drug toxicity (e.g., carbamazepine can worsen myoclonic seizures; clobazam can increase simple partial seizures; vigabatrin can worsen absences)

Other Therapies

- Consider epilepsy surgery *early* in intractable cases that have not responded to two first-line agents and one add-on agent, that have been evaluated for other factors possibly contributing to intractability, and that meet the criteria (including focal origin of epilepsy or atonic attacks) discussed in Chapter 9.
- An implanted, battery-powered stimulator attached to the vagus nerve in the neck is a new form of epilepsy therapy that has significantly reduced seizures in about one-third of patients with little morbidity. It is presently used in some intractable patients who are not candidates for conventional intracranial surgery (see Chapter 9).

- Patients who are resistant to or cannot tolerate standard AEDs and are not surgical candidates may benefit from entry into a clinical trial with an AED in development.

Suggested Reading

Pharmacokinetics and Mechanisms

Bourgeois BFD. Important pharmacokinetic properties of AEDs. Epilepsia 1995;36(Suppl 5):S1-S7.

Cloyd J. Pharmacokinetic pitfalls of present antiepileptic medications. Epilepsia 1991;32 (Suppl 5):S53-S65.

Graves NM. Neuropharmacology and drug interactions in clinical practice. Epilepsia 1995;36(Suppl 2):S27-S33.

Kupferberg HJ, Schmutz M. Screening of New Compounds and the Role of the Pharmaceutical Industry. In J Engel Jr, TA Pedley (eds), Epilepsy: A Comprehensive Textbook. New York: Lippincott-Raven, 1998;1417-1434.

Macdonald RL, Greenfield LJ. Mechanisms of action of new AEDs. Curr Opin Neurol 1997;10:121-128.

Meldrum B. Update on the mechanism of action of AEDs. Epilepsia 1996;37(Suppl 6): S4-S11.

Patsalos PN, Duncan JS. Anti-epileptic drugs: a review of clinically significant drug interactions. Drug Safety 1993;9:156-184.

White HS. Mechanisms of Action of Antiepileptic Drugs. In RJ Porter, D Chadwick (eds), The Epilepsies 2. Boston: Butterworth-Heinemann, 1997;1-30.

White HS, Woodhead JH, Franklin MR, et al. General Principles. Experimental Selection, Quantification, and Evaluation of Anti-Epileptic Drugs. In RH Levy, RH Mattson, BS Meldrum, et al. (eds), Anti-Epileptic Drugs (4th ed). New York: Raven, 1995;99-110.

Willmore LJ. The effect of age on pharmacokinetics of anti-epileptic drugs. Epilepsia 1995;36(Suppl 5):S14-S21.

Treatment Principles

Asconapé JJ, Penry JK. Use of AEDs in the presence of liver and kidney diseases: a review. Epilepsia 1982;23(Suppl 1):S65-S79.

Britton JW, So EL. Selection of AEDs: a practical approach. Mayo Clin Proc 1996;71:778-786.

Brodie MJ. Drug interactions in epilepsy. Epilepsia 1992;33(Suppl 1):S13-S22.

Chadwick D. Rational Drug Therapy for Epilepsy. In RJ Porter, D Chadwick (eds), The Epilepsies 2. Boston: Butterworth-Heinemann, 1997;247-266.

Chadwick D, Reynolds EH. When do epileptic patients need treatment? Starting and stopping medication. BMJ 1985;290:1885-1888.

Deckers CLP, Hekster YA, Keyser A, et al. Reappraisal of polytherapy in epilepsy: a critical review of drug load and adverse effects. Epilepsia 1997;38:570-575.

Duncan JS, Patsalos PN, Shorvon SD. Effects of discontinuation of phenytoin, carbamazepine and valproate on concomitant antiepileptic medication. Epilepsia 1991;32:101-116.

Gilmore RL. Seizures and antiepileptic drug use in transplant patients. Neurol Clin 1988;6:274-296.

Graves NM. Neuropharmacology and drug interactions in clinical practice. Epilepsia 1995;36(Suppl 2):S27-S33.

Graves NM, Leppik IE. Advances in pharmacotherapy: recent developments in the treatment of epilepsy. J Clin Pharmacol Therap 1993;18:227-242.
Leppik IE. Metabolism of antiepileptic medication: newborn to elderly. Epilepsia 1992;33(Suppl 4):S32-S40.
Levy RH, Koch KM. Drug interactions with valproic acid. Drugs 1982;24:543-556.
Macdonald RL. Seizure Disorders and Epilepsy. In MV Johnston, RL Macdonald, AB Young (eds), Principles of Drug Therapy in Neurology. Philadelphia: F. A. Davis, 1991;87-117.
Macdonald RL, Richens A. Rational polypharmacy. Seizure 1995;4:211-214.
Mattson RH. The role of the old and the new AEDs in special populations: mental and multiple handicaps. Epilepsia 1996;37(Suppl 6):S45-S53.
Perucca E. Pharmacological principles as a basis for polytherapy. Acta Neurol Scand 1995;162:31-34.
Reynolds EH, Shorvon SD. Monotherapy or polytherapy for epilepsy? Epilepsia 1981;22:1-10.
Richens A. Rational polypharmacy. Seizure 1995;4:211-214.
Theodore WH, Porter RJ. Removal of sedative-hypnotic antiepileptics from the regimens of patients with intractable epilepsy. Ann Neurol 1983;13:320-324.
Wilder BJ. Treatment considerations in anticonvulsant monotherapy. Epilepsia 1987;28 (Suppl 2):S1-S7.
Zahn CA, Morrell MJ, Collins SD, et al. Management issues for women with epilepsy. A review of the literature. Neurology 1998;51:949-956.

Serum Levels of Antiepileptic Drugs

Commission on Anti-Epileptic Drugs of the ILAE. Guidelines for therapeutic monitoring of anti-epileptic drugs. Epilepsia 1993;34:585-587.
Eadie MJ. Plasma antiepileptic drug monitoring in a neurological practice: a 25 year experience. Ther Drug Monitor 1994;16:458-468.
Eadie MJ. The role of therapeutic drug monitoring in improving the cost effectiveness of anticonvulsant therapy. Clin Pharmacokinet 1995;29:29-35.
Mattson RH. Antiepileptic drug monitoring: a reappraisal. Epilepsia 1995;36(Suppl 5):S22-S29.
Rosenthal E, Hoffer E, Ben-Aryeh H, et al. Use of saliva in home monitoring of carbamazepine levels. Epilepsia 1995;36:72-74.

Ketogenic Diet

Ballaban-Gil K, Callahan C, O'Dell C, et al. Complications of the ketogenic diet. Epilepsia 1998;39:744-748.
Kinsman SL, Vining EP, Quaskey SA, et al. Efficacy of the ketogenic diet for intractable seizure disorders: a review of 58 cases. Epilepsia 1992;33:1132-1136.
Nordli DR Jr, DeVivo DC. The ketogenic diet revisited: back to the future. Epilepsia 1997;38:743-749.

6 Individual Antiepileptic Drugs

Carbamazepine (Tegretol, Tegretol-XR, Carbatrol, Tegretol CR in Canada)

Chemical Features

- Tricyclic compound
- Iminodibenzyl ring structure

Mechanism of Action

- Reduces voltage and use-dependent, sustained, high-frequency, repetitive firing of neurons
- Produces a voltage and use-dependent blockade of sodium channels
- Stabilizes neural membranes
- Reduces synaptic transmission

Pharmacology

- Absorption
  - Slow and erratic.
  - Bioavailability is 75–85%.
  - Average time to peak concentration is 2–8 hours.
  - Administration with food has a variable effect but is of little clinical significance.
- Protein binding
  - Seventy-five percent to 80% is bound to albumin and alpha-acid glycoprotein.
  - Protein binding interactions are not clinically significant.
- Half-life
  - 5–12 hours.
  - As with other AEDs, the half-life of carbamazepine is age dependent.
- Therapeutic range
  - The therapeutic range is wide: 4–12 μg/ml (20–50 μmol/liter).
  - A large intersubject variability exists.
- Drug interactions
  - Carbamazepine induces its own metabolism (autoinduction). After several weeks or a few months of therapy, the dosage may need to be increased to maintain satisfactory seizure control.

  - Higher plasma concentrations occur with the concurrent use of erythromycin, clarithromycin (Biaxin), fluoxetine, propoxyphene, cimetidine, diltiazem, danazol, and isoniazid.
  - Lower plasma concentrations occur with concurrent use of other hepatic-inducing AEDs, such as primidone, phenobarbital, phenytoin, and felbamate.
  - Carbamazepine's induction of cytochrome P450 3A4 (CYP3A4) results in decreased levels of oral contraceptive hormones and cyclosporin. The metabolism of warfarin (Coumadin), tricyclic antidepressants, clozapine, haloperidol, theophylline, doxycycline, ethosuximide, lamotrigine, topiramate, felbamate, and tiagabine is also enhanced.
  - The effect of carbamazepine on the clearance of other AEDs is variable.
- Elimination
  - Carbamazepine is predominantly eliminated by hepatic metabolism.
  - The major metabolic product is carbamazepine 10,11-epoxide.
  - CYP3A4 frequently catalyzes this reaction.
  - Carbamazepine 10,11-epoxide may be responsible for some of the clinical efficacy and toxicity of carbamazepine.
  - Hepatic enzyme induction results in higher carbamazepine 10,11-epoxide levels.
  - Valproate may increase the carbamazepine 10,11-epoxide to carbamazepine ratio, but the mechanism has not been defined.

Daily Dose

- Adults: 600–1,200 mg.
- Children: 10–30 mg/kg.
- Therapy can be initiated in children with 100 mg once or twice a day and in adults with 200 mg once or twice a day.
- Carbamazepine is generally administered in three divided doses. The controlled-release formulation can be administered twice a day.

Efficacy

- Tonic-clonic seizures
- Partial seizures

Principal Adverse Effects

- Dose-related
  - Diplopia, headaches, dizziness, ataxia, gastrointestinal upset, tremors, fatigue, incoordination, drowsiness
  - Worsening of certain seizures, especially myoclonic
- Idiosyncratic/allergic
  - Skin rashes in 5–15%; rarely Stevens-Johnson syndrome or hypersensitivity syndrome.
  - Drug-induced lupus is rare.

  - Hepatic/hematologic toxicity or pancreatitis is rare.
- Chronic
  - Transient, mild leucopenia can occur in 5–20% of patients.
  - Hyponatremia due to syndrome of inappropriate secretion of antidiuretic hormone (SIADH); usually not clinically significant.
  - Cardiac conduction disturbances are rare and most often observed in older patients.
  - May exacerbate seizures, most frequently myoclonic or atypical absence seizures.
  - Cognitive impairment occurs in some patients.
  - Effect on vitamin D and calcium metabolism is generally less than with phenytoin.
  - Behavioral changes are uncommon.
  - Movement disorders are rare.
- Teratogenicity
  - Minor anomalies and major malformations have been observed, as with other AEDs.
  - Some studies suggest that carbamazepine may be less teratogenic than phenytoin or primidone.
  - Incidence of spina bifida is 0.5%.
  - Teratogenic potential increases when carbamazepine is used in polytherapy.

Advantages

- Nonsedating in therapeutic range
- Twice-daily dosing with extended-release formulation
- May be less teratogenic than most other agents
- Relatively low cost

Disadvantages

- Neurotoxic above a narrow therapeutic range
- Limited spectrum of efficacy
- Neurotoxicity common during initiation of therapeutic doses
- Idiosyncratic reactions relatively common (e.g., skin rash that is rarely severe)
- No parenteral form available
- May exacerbate seizures (especially myoclonic)
- Potential cognitive toxicity
- Microsomal enzyme inducer

Clobazam (Frisium)

Chemical Features

- A 1,5-benzodiazepine
- Poorly water soluble

Mechanism of Action

- Similar to other benzodiazepines (see Clonazepam, later)

Pharmacology

- Absorption
  - Well absorbed.
  - Time to peak concentration is 1–4 hours.
  - Food has variable effect on absorption.
- Protein binding
  - 85%.
  - Protein-binding interactions can occur but generally are not clinically significant.
- Half-life
  - 10–30 hours.
  - Half-life of active metabolite *N*-desmethyl clobazam ranges from 35 to 50 hours.
  - Half-life increases with age.
- Drug interactions
  - Interaction with other AEDs is variable.
  - Can rarely cause an increase in the plasma concentration of phenytoin, carbamazepine, valproate, and phenobarbital.
  - Cimetidine and alcohol may cause increase of clobazam concentration.
  - Hepatic enzyme-inducing AEDs may increase the *N*-desmethyl clobazam-to-clobazam ratio.
- Elimination
  - Extensively metabolized to a number of compounds.
  - *N*-Desmethyl clobazam is the most important active metabolite.
  - Well metabolized by children and adults.
  - Elimination reduced in cases with severe liver disease.

Daily Dose

- Adults: 20–60 mg.
- Children: 0.5–2.0 mg/kg.
- In adults, therapy should be initiated with a single 5- to 10-mg dose at bedtime.
- In children, the initial dose should be 5 mg per day.

Efficacy

- Similar to other benzodiazepines, but generally better tolerated.
- The benzodiazepine of choice.
- Most frequently used as adjunctive therapy in the treatment of primary generalized and partial seizure disorders, including Lennox-Gastaut syndrome.

- Can be used intermittently in the treatment of seizures associated with the menstrual cycle.
- Can be effective in partial or nonconvulsive generalized status epilepticus given as a loading dose of 60–70 mg in adults.
- Tolerance develops in approximately 50% of excellent responders and in 30% of responders overall.

Principal Adverse Effects

- Dose-related
  - Drowsiness, dizziness, fatigue, ataxia, irritability, depression, impotence, hypersalivation.
  - Side effects are usually mild.
  - Can exacerbate seizures, especially simple partial.
- Idiosyncratic/allergic: rare skin rash
- Chronic
  - Sedation.
  - Withdrawal may precipitate seizures.
- Teratogenicity: none known

Advantages

- Broad spectrum
- Well tolerated
- No long-term cognitive or tissue side effects
- Rapid onset of effect
- Once or twice daily dosing
- Favorable pharmacokinetics
- No hepatic enzyme induction
- Rare interactions with other AEDs
- Serum levels not required
- Antianxiety effect
- Appears effective in monotherapy
- Relatively inexpensive
- Potentially low teratogenicity

Disadvantages

- Tolerance (in at least 20–30% overall and in 50% of excellent responders)
- Drowsiness common
- Occasional behavioral side effects
- May exacerbate seizures in some patients
- No parenteral preparation
- May produce withdrawal effects on cessation of therapy, including seizure worsening

Clonazepam (Klonopin, Rivotril in Canada)

Chemical Features

- A 1,4-benzodiazepine
- A chlorinated derivative of nitrazepam

Mechanism of Action

- Enhances GABA-ergic transmission
- Acts at benzodiazepine binding sites of $GABA_A$ receptor complex
- Increases $GABA_A$ receptor opening frequency, which results in increased chloride uptake and hyperpolarization

Pharmacology

- Absorption
  - More than 80% bioavailability.
  - Peak concentration is reached 1–4 hours after oral administration.
- Protein binding: 85%
- Half-life: 20–70 hours
- Therapeutic range: poor correlation between plasma concentration and clinical efficacy
- Drug interactions
  - Carbamazepine, phenobarbital, and primidone may lower clonazepam concentration.
  - Phenytoin has a variable effect.
  - May cause respiratory depression when used with barbiturates.
  - May cause absence status when used with valproate.
- Elimination: almost completely eliminated by hepatic metabolism to inactive metabolites

Daily Dose

- Adults: 2–6 mg.
- Children 0.1–0.2 mg/kg.
- Initiate therapy in adults with 0.5 mg tid.
- Initiate therapy in children with 0.5 mg daily. Increase by 0.5-mg increments.

Efficacy

- Most frequently used as adjunctive therapy in the treatment of both primary generalized and partial seizure disorders, including Lennox-Gastaut syndrome.
- Tolerance occurs in up to 50% of patients who respond.

Principal Adverse Effects

- Dose-related
  - Drowsiness, ataxia, behavioral and personality changes. Other neurologic side effects are less common.
  - Appearance of other seizure types.
  - Increased frequency of seizures.
- Idiosyncratic/allergic: leukopenia rare
- Chronic
  - Sedation.
  - Peripheral edema.
  - Cognitive.
  - Withdrawal may precipitate seizures.
- Teratogenicity: minimal

Ethosuximide (Zarontin)

Chemical Properties

- A substituted succinimide with a ring structure that resembles phenytoin
- Water soluble

Mechanism of Action

- Reduces voltage-dependent, low-threshold calcium current in thalamic neurons

Pharmacology

- Absorption
  - Well absorbed.
  - Time to reach peak concentration is 1–6 hours.
- Protein binding: negligible
- Half-life
  - 40–60 hours in adults
  - 30–40 hours in children
- Therapeutic range: Best control generally achieved with plasma concentrations in the range of 40–100 μg/ml (350–700 μmol/liter), but drug regimen has to be individualized. Higher levels may be necessary for optimal control in some patients.
- Drug interactions
  - Hepatic enzyme-inducting AEDs increase the clearance of ethosuximide.
  - Interactions are generally minor.
  - No interactions with oral contraceptives.

- Elimination
  - Eliminated by hepatic metabolism
  - 20% excreted unchanged in the urine

Daily Dose

- Adults: 1,000–2,000 mg.
- Children: 15–40 mg/kg.
- In adults, initiate therapy with 500 mg a day and increase by 250-mg increments.
- In children, initiate therapy with 250 mg daily and increase by 250-mg increments.

Efficacy

- Absence seizures.
- Typical absence seizures respond better than atypical absences.

Principal Adverse Effects

- Dose-related: drowsiness, fatigue, headache, hiccups, nausea, depression
- Idiosyncratic/allergic
  - Reactions are rare.
  - Skin rash.
  - Pancytopenia.
  - Lupus-like syndrome.
- Chronic
  - Minimal
  - Exacerbation of absence seizures
- Teratogenicity: none known

Advantages

- Well tolerated
- Minimal drug interactions
- No known teratogenicity

Disadvantages

- Narrow spectrum
- Occasional gastrointestinal upset

Felbamate (Felbatol)

Chemical Features

- A dicarbamate

- Chemically related to meprobamate
- Poorly water soluble

Mechanism of Action

- Facilitates GABA-ergic transmission
- Blocks NMDA responses

Pharmacology

- Absorption
  - Well absorbed
  - Peak concentration reached in 2-6 hours
  - Not affected by food
- Protein binding: not significant
- Half-life
  - 13-23 hours
  - Shorter half-life in children
- Therapeutic range
  - Not well established.
  - In adult clinical trials, better response was observed with plasma concentration of 60-80 μg/ml.
- Drug interactions
  - Can cause an increase in the plasma concentration of valproate, phenobarbital, phenytoin, carbamazepine epoxide.
  - Decreases plasma concentration of carbamazepine.
  - Hepatic enzyme-inducing AEDs increase clearance.
- Elimination
  - Eliminated by hepatic metabolism and partly by renal excretion.
  - Metabolites are not clinically active.
  - Well metabolized by children and adults.

Daily Dose

- Adults: up to 3,600 mg.
- Children: up to 45 mg/kg.
- A slow titration schedule is recommended.
- Can initiate therapy in adults with 400 mg tid with dose increases every 1-2 weeks.
- In children, can initiate therapy with 15 mg/kg.

Efficacy

- Clinical trials demonstrated efficacy against partial and generalized tonic-clonic seizures and various seizure types associated with the Lennox-Gastaut syndrome.

Principal Adverse Effects

- Dose-related: nausea and vomiting, headache, anorexia, weight loss, blurred vision, ataxia, insomnia
- Idiosyncratic/allergic
  - Hypersensitivity reactions in up to 4% of patients
  - Aplastic anemia (may be fatal) reported in 27 patients worldwide
  - Liver failure (may be fatal) reported in 14 patients worldwide
- Chronic
  - None known.
  - No cognitive side effects.
  - Some patients report increased alertness.
- Teratogenicity: teratogenic potential unknown

Advantages

- Long half-life
- Twice daily dosing in adults
- Serum levels not required
- Efficacy against a variety of seizure types, including Lennox-Gastaut syndrome
- Well tolerated by majority of patients
- May have an alerting effect

Disadvantages

- Rare but serious idiosyncratic hematologic and hepatic toxicity
- Drug interactions
- No parenteral formulation
- Relatively expensive compared with traditional AEDs
- Slow titration
- Teratogenicity unknown

Gabapentin (Neurontin)

Chemical Features

- A structural analog of GABA
- Highly water soluble

Mechanism of Action

- Major effect responsible for antiepileptic properties remains to be elucidated.
- In animal models, after intravenous administration, peak effect is delayed for approximately 2 hours, past the time of maximal plasma concentration.

- No effect on $GABA_A$ receptor.
- Increases rate of GABA synthesis.
- Elevates brain GABA levels.
- Effect on L-amino acid transport system.
- Novel binding site in central nervous system (CNS).

Pharmacology

- Absorption
  - Uses L-amino acid transport system.
  - Absorption is saturable and dose dependent: 60% absorption with 300-mg dose, 35% with 4,800-mg dose (1,600 mg tid).
  - Bioavailability can be increased by increasing the frequency of dosing.
  - Administration with food does not alter absorption.
  - Peak plasma concentration achieved after 2–3 hours.
- Protein binding: none
- Half-life
  - 5–8 hours
  - Increased half-life in older patients
- Therapeutic range: not established
- Drug interactions
  - No significant drug interactions have been identified except reduced renal clearance of felbamate.
  - Antacids may cause a slight decrease in absorption.
  - No interaction with oral contraceptives.

Daily Dose

- Adults: 1,200–4,200 mg.
- Children: 30–60 mg/kg.
- In adults, can initiate therapy with 300 mg on first day, 300 mg bid on day 2, and 300 mg tid on day 3. Further dose increases can be made according to response.
- In children, can initiate therapy with 20–30 mg/kg.

Efficacy

- Adjunctive therapy in partial and secondarily generalized seizures

Principal Adverse Effects

- Dose-related: drowsiness, dizziness, fatigue, ataxia, myoclonus
- Idiosyncratic/allergic: rare
- Chronic
  - Weight gain
  - No cognitive side effects

- Teratogenicity
  - None reported
  - Teratogenic potential unknown

Advantages

- Very well tolerated
- Favorable pharmacokinetics (not metabolized)
- No drug interactions
- Rapid titration possible
- No long-term tissue or cognitive side effects
- Serum level monitoring not required
- Potential low teratogenicity

Disadvantages

- Three times daily dosing
- Fairly narrow spectrum of efficacy
- Moderate bioavailability
- Relatively expensive compared with traditional AEDs
- No parenteral preparation

Lamotrigine (Lamictal)

Chemical Features

- A triazine derivative
- Water soluble

Mechanism of Action

- Use-dependent blocker of voltage-gated sodium channels
- Reduces discharge frequency of rapidly firing neurons
- May inhibit pathologic release of the excitatory amino acids glutamate and aspartate
- Weak, insignificant antifolate effect

Pharmacology

- Absorption
  - Almost complete bioavailability.
  - Food does not alter absorption.
  - Peak plasma concentration achieved in 2–4 hours.
- Protein binding
  - 55%
  - No protein-binding interactions
- Half-life
  - In volunteers, as monotherapy: 24–30 hours

- In presence of hepatic enzyme inducers such as phenytoin, carbamazepine, phenobarbital, primidone: 15 hours
- In presence of valproate: 48-60 hours
- In presence of valproate plus an enzyme-inducing AED: 24-30 hours
- Therapeutic range: not established
- Drug interactions
  - Valproate inhibits elimination.
  - Hepatic enzyme-inducing AEDs increase elimination.
  - Pharmacodynamic interaction with carbamazepine.
  - No interaction with oral contraceptives.
- Elimination
  - Metabolized by first-order kinetics to inactive metabolites
  - Considerable intersubject variability

Daily Dose

- Lamotrigine dose schedule

Adjunctive Therapy in Children

	With Hepatic Enzyme-Inducing AEDs		
Treatment Week	*Without Valproate*	*With Valproate*	*Valproate Alone*
1 and 2	2 mg/kg	1 mg/kg	0.15 mg/kg
3 and 4	5 mg/kg	2.5 mg/kg	0.30 mg/kg
Maintenance	5-15 mg/kg	5-10 mg/kg	1-15 mg/kg

Adjunctive Therapy in Adults

	With Hepatic Enzyme-Inducing AEDs		
Treatment Week	*Without Valproate*	*With Valproate*	*Valproate Alone*
1 and 2	50 mg once a day	25 mg once a day	12.5 mg daily
3 and 4	50 mg bid	25 mg bid	25 mg once a day
Maintenance	250-300 mg bid	150-200 mg bid	50-100 mg bid

Monotherapy

	Adults	*Children*
Weeks 1 and 2	25 mg	0.5 mg/kg
Weeks 3 and 4	25 mg bid	1 mg/kg
Maintenance	50-100 mg bid	2-8 mg/kg

Efficacy

- Adjunctive therapy in the treatment of primary generalized seizures (tonic-clonic, myoclonic, absence, atonic, tonic) and partial seizures.
- Lennox-Gastaut syndrome.
- Monotherapy can be achieved in some patients.

Principal Adverse Effects

- Dose-related: fatigue, diplopia, headache, ataxia, dizziness, drowsiness, nystagmus, insomnia
- Idiosyncratic/allergic
  - Rash in 5–10%.
  - Serious rash in 1%.
  - Rash is more common in children.
  - *Stevens-Johnson syndrome*; or rarely its more severe form, toxic epidermal necrolysis; or AED hypersensitivity syndrome occurs in up to one of 100 children and one of 1,000 adults on the drug. The vast majority of severe skin rashes occurs in the first 8 weeks of therapy.
  - Data suggest that the incidence of rash and severe rash increases with valproate cotherapy and initial doses or dosage escalation exceeding manufacturer's recommendations.
  - Careful monitoring and discontinuation if there is no alternative explanation for the rash are indicated if a rash develops.
- Chronic: none reported
- Teratogenicity
  - None reported
  - Teratogenic potential unknown

Advantages

- Broad spectrum
- Favorable pharmacokinetics (once or twice a day dosage)
- Serum levels not required
- No long-term tissue or cognitive side effects
- Appears effective in monotherapy
- Is not an enzyme inducer
- Potential low teratogenicity

Disadvantages

- Skin rash in 5–10%; rarely serious
- Very slow titration
- $T_{1/2}$ affected by other AEDs
- Relatively expensive compared with traditional AEDs
- No parenteral preparation

Oxcarbazepine (Trileptal)

Chemical Features

- The keto analog of carbamazepine
- Low water solubility

Mechanism of Action

- Probably similar to that of carbamazepine.
- Sodium channel blocker.
- Anticonvulsant activity is predominantly related to its active metabolite 10,11-dihydro-10-hydroxy-5H-dibenzazepine-5-carboxamide (MHD), to which it is almost completely converted.

Pharmacology

- Absorption: almost complete
- Protein binding
  - 60%
  - 40% (MHD metabolite)
- Half-life (MHD)
  - Oxcarbazepine is rapidly and almost completely converted to MHD.
  - Half-life of MHD: 8–10 hours.
  - No autoinduction.
- Therapeutic range
  - Not well established.
  - Levels of 50–130 μmol/liter have been suggested.
- Drug interactions
  - Less than with carbamazepine.
  - May cause slight elevation of valproate or phenytoin levels.
  - Barbiturates and phenytoin decrease serum concentration of MHD.
  - May induce the metabolism of estrogen in oral contraceptives, increasing the contraceptive failure rate.
  - No interaction with erythromycin or oral anticoagulants.
- Elimination
  - Almost completely metabolized to MHD.
  - No epoxide is formed.
  - Metabolites excreted by the kidney.
  - 1% unchanged.

Daily dose

- Adults: 900–3,600 mg
- Children: mean 30–40 mg/kg

Efficacy

- Partial seizures
- Tonic-clonic seizures

Principal Adverse Effects

- Dose-related
  - Dizziness, ataxia, headaches, fatigue

  - Incidence of side effects lower than with carbamazepine
  - No cognitive effect
- Idiosyncratic/allergic
  - Allergic skin reactions occur less frequently than with carbamazepine.
  - Cross-reactivity in patients with carbamazepine-induced skin rash occurs in approximately 25% of cases.
- Chronic
  - Hyponatremia more common than with carbamazepine.
  - Systemic side effects are rare.
- Teratogenicity: teratogenic potential unknown

Advantages

- Fewer drug interactions than with carbamazepine.
- No autoinduction.
- No epoxide metabolite.
- Fewer allergic reactions than with carbamazepine.
- Incidence of dose-related side effects is less than with carbamazepine.

Disadvantages

- Higher incidence of hyponatremia than with carbamazepine
- No parenteral formulation
- Teratogenic potential unknown

Phenobarbital

Chemical Features

- A substituted barbituric acid.
- Low aqueous solubility.
- Sodium salt is freely water soluble.

Mechanism of Action

- Suppresses discharge of epileptic foci
- Binds to $GABA_A$ receptor complex
- Facilitates inhibition by GABA by prolonging chloride channel opening time
- Sodium channel blocker

Pharmacology

- Absorption
  - High bioavailability.

- Average time to peak concentration is 2 hours.
- Administration with food does not alter bioavailability.
- Protein binding
  - 50%
  - No significant protein-binding interactions
- Half-life
  - 25–150 hours.
  - Newborns have longest half-life.
- Therapeutic range
  - 20–40 μg/ml (80–200 μmol/liter).
  - Value of measuring plasma levels is limited because of large variability.
- Drug interactions
  - Both competitive inhibitor and inducer of hepatic enzymes.
  - Interaction with phenytoin is variable.
  - Valproate reduces phenobarbital elimination.
  - Carbamazepine, benzodiazepines usually do not alter phenobarbital level.
  - No interaction with vigabatrin, gabapentin.
  - Phenobarbital enhances hepatic clearance of oral contraceptives, steroids, antibiotics, psychotropics, tricyclic antidepressants, calcium channel blockers, theophylline, digitoxin, acetaminophen, cimetidine, cyclosporin, lamotrigine, felbamate, topiramate, tiagabine.
- Elimination
  - Eliminated both by hepatic metabolism and pH-dependent renal excretion.
  - Eliminated by first-order kinetics.
  - Influenced by age, diuresis, urinary pH (increased excretion with alkaline pH), drug interactions.
  - Elimination is impaired in advanced renal disease and may be reduced in presence of hepatic disease.

Daily Dose

- Adults: 90–250 mg.
- Children: 2–5 mg/kg.
- Total daily dose can be administered once a day at bedtime.

Efficacy

- Tonic-clonic, partial, and neonatal seizures
- Parenterally in the treatment of convulsive status epilepticus
- Although rarely indicated, is effective for prophylaxis of febrile seizures

Principal Adverse Effects

- Dose-related: drowsiness, blurred vision, ataxia, fatigue, dizziness, depression
- Idiosyncratic/allergic: skin rash in 5–10%

- Chronic
  - Cognitive impairment, behavioral disturbances, decreased concentration.
  - Abrupt discontinuation can result in withdrawal symptoms.
  - Affects vitamin D and calcium metabolism (osteomalacia).
  - Megaloblastic changes.
  - Interferes with vitamin K–dependent clotting factors in fetus.
  - Connective tissue changes (muscle aches and pains, frozen shoulder, Dupuytren's contracture, Peyronie's syndrome, Ledderhose syndrome).
- Teratogenicity
  - Gross malformations are less common than with other AEDs.
  - Dysmorphic features can occur as with other AEDs.
  - Changes in neural development with reduced head circumference.
  - Reduced birth weight.

Advantages

- Low cost
- Once daily dosing
- Relatively broad spectrum
- Parenteral form available

Disadvantages

- Sedating
- Long-term cognitive, memory, and behavioral effects
- Occasional long-term connective tissue effects
- Withdrawal effects
- Teratogenic
- Microsomal enzyme inducer

Primidone (Mysoline)

Chemical Features

- Chemically, is deoxyphenobarbital
- Poorly water soluble

Mechanism of Action

- Activity related to primidone itself and its metabolite, phenobarbital.
- Phenylethylmalonamide (PEMA) metabolite does not play a major role.
- Similar to phenobarbital.
- Synergistic effect with phenobarbital.

Pharmacology

- Absorption
  - Well absorbed.

- Average time to peak concentration is 3–4 hours.
- Administration with food does not reduce bioavailability.
- Protein binding: no significant protein binding
- Half-life
  - 10–25 hours, mean 12 hours
  - Shorter in patients on polytherapy with other hepatic enzyme-inducing AEDs
  - Influenced by age and drug interactions
- Therapeutic range
  - 3–8 μg/ml (15–40 μmol/liter).
  - Value of measuring plasma concentration is limited.
  - Long-term therapy correlates better with phenobarbital levels.
  - Important to monitor phenobarbital levels.
- Drug interactions
  - Synergistic effect with phenobarbital.
  - Higher phenobarbital to primidone blood level ratios in patients on polytherapy with hepatic enzyme-inducing AEDs.
  - Valproate increases primidone levels.
  - Reduces effect of steroids and oral contraceptives.
  - Reduced anticoagulant effect with Coumadin.
- Elimination
  - Metabolized to phenobarbital and phenylethylmalonamide.
  - Age-dependent.
  - Increased clearance during pregnancy.
  - Renal disease and hepatic disease may reduce clearance.

Daily Dose

- Adults: 750–1,000 mg.
- Children: 5–20 mg/kg.
- Initiate therapy in adults with 125 mg at bedtime for several days; increase dose in 125-mg increments.
- Children can be started on one-half the adult dose.
- Should be administered in three times daily dosing.

Efficacy

- Tonic-clonic seizures
- Partial seizures
- Some efficacy against myoclonic seizures

Principal Adverse Effects

- Similar to phenobarbital; generally less well tolerated
- Dose-related: drowsiness, ataxia, blurred vision, dizziness, fatigue, depression
- Idiosyncratic/allergic: skin rash in 5–10%
- Chronic

  - Cognitive impairment
  - Sexual dysfunction
  - Connective tissue disorders
  - Effect on vitamin D and calcium metabolism
- Teratogenicity: similar to phenobarbital and phenytoin

Phenytoin (Dilantin)

Chemical Features

- Available as free acid and sodium salt
- Contains a hydantoin ring
- Poorly water soluble

Mechanism of Action

- Membrane stabilizer
- Blocks post-tetanic potentiation
- Impairs sustained repetitive firing of neurons
- Causes use-dependent blockage of sodium channels

Pharmacology

- Absorption
  - Well absorbed with 85–90% bioavailability.
  - Average time to peak concentration is 4–8 hours.
  - Poorly absorbed by newborns.
  - Absorption may be decreased by antacids and enteral feedings.
  - Administration with food does not reduce bioavailability.
- Protein binding
  - 75–95% protein binding, generally 90–95%
  - Significant protein-binding interactions with other protein-bound drugs and endogenous hormones
  - Decreased protein-binding during pregnancy and in the presence of hepatic or renal disease and other hypoalbuminemic states
- Half-life
  - Because of elimination by saturation (zero-order) kinetics, apparent half-life is dose dependent.
  - 8–40 hours, generally 20–24 hours.
  - Longer half-life in neonates.
  - Shorter half-life in children.
  - Half-life shortened by coadministration with other hepatic enzyme–inducing AEDs.

- Therapeutic range
  - Large intersubject variability.
  - 10–20 μg/ml (40–80 μmol/liter).
  - Patients who have lower protein binding (e.g., uremia) may be well controlled at lower plasma concentrations because of higher free fraction.
- Drug interactions
  - Interactions are common.
  - Protein-binding interactions can occur with salicylate, phenylbutazone, tolbutamide, and valproate.
  - Antacids may impair absorption.
  - Higher plasma concentrations can be seen during concurrent administration of isoniazid, disulfiram, tolbutamide, allopurinol, cimetidine, chloramphenicol, warfarin, sulfonamides, and diltiazem.
  - Lower plasma concentrations can be seen with the concurrent administration or use of vigabatrin (20% decrease in phenytoin), ethanol, and antineoplastic drugs such as cisplatin, vinblastine, bleomycin, and rifampin.
  - Benzodiazepine, carbamazepine, and phenobarbital effect is variable.
  - Phenytoin reduces the efficacy of a number of drugs, including Coumadin; steroids and oral contraceptives; antibiotics such as chloramphenicol; and cyclosporin, theophylline, digitoxin, quinidine, meperidine, furosemide, praziquantel, carbamazepine, lamotrigine, topiramate, felbamate, and tiagabine.
  - Phenytoin accentuates vitamin D and calcium metabolism and vitamin K-dependent clotting factors.
- Elimination
  - Phenytoin is extensively and almost completely metabolized through an arene oxide intermediate.
  - Cytochrome P450 isoforms of the CYP2C subgroup are responsible for parahydroxylation of phenytoin.
  - Eliminated by zero-order kinetics.
  - Metabolism is slow in neonates and enhanced in children; it may decrease slightly in advanced age. It is influenced by concurrent drug therapy.

Daily Dose

- Adults: 300–400 mg.
- Children: 4–8 mg/kg.
- Dose must be individualized according to patient's response and side effects.
- Can be administered to adults once a day.
- Therapy can be initiated in adults with 300 mg daily; children can be initiated with 4 mg/kg daily.
- Phenytoin sodium capsules contain 8% less phenytoin than tablets (free acid).
- Because of its saturation kinetics, phenytoin in the higher dose ranges should be increased by 30- to 50-mg increments to avoid toxicity.

Efficacy

- Tonic-clonic seizures
- Partial seizures
- Status epilepticus

Principal Adverse Effects

- Dose-related: nystagmus, cerebellovestibular, drowsiness, fatigue, dysarthria, tremors, impaired concentration, encephalopathy
- Idiosyncratic/allergic
  - Skin allergy in 5–10% of patients
  - Immunologic, vasculitis, hematologic (all rare)
- Chronic: may involve several systems—neurologic, connective tissue, dermatologic, endocrine, metabolic—and deficiency states
  - Neurologic: peripheral neuropathy, cognitive and behavioral side effects
  - Connective tissue: coarsened facial features, gingival hyperplasia, pulmonary fibrosis, Dupuytren's contracture
  - Dermatologic: acne, hirsutism
  - Endocrine: changes in the protein binding of sex steroids, thyroid hormones, metabolic bone changes (hypocalcemia and osteomalacia)
  - Hematologic: folate deficiency (generally not clinically significant), neonatal coagulation defects, megaloblastic changes
- Teratogenicity
  - Minor anomalies and major malformations described as with other AEDs.
  - Although a fetal hydantoin syndrome has been described, similar anomalies have been observed with other AEDs.

Advantages

- Nonsedating in therapeutic range
- Long half-life (once-daily dose)
- Parenteral preparation
- Low cost
- Multiple oral formulations
- Loading or rapid titration possible

Disadvantages

- Neurotoxic above a narrow therapeutic range
- Limited spectrum of efficacy
- Connective tissue and other cosmetic changes
- Other long-term tissue and cognitive toxicity
- Saturation kinetics
- Microsomal enzyme inducer
- Teratogenic

Tiagabine (Gabitril)

Chemical Features

- A nipecotic acid derivative
- Poorly water soluble

Mechanism of Action

- Blocks reuptake of GABA into neurons and glia through the GABA transporter and thus enhances GABA-ergic transmission

Pharmacology

- Absorption
  - Well absorbed.
  - Peak concentration reached in 2 hours.
  - Food delays the absorption rate but not its extent.
- Protein binding: 95%
- Half-life
  - 4–8 hours (as monotherapy)
  - Shorter when used with hepatic enzyme–inducing AEDs (2–3 hours)
- Therapeutic range: not well-established

Drug Interactions

- Hepatic enzyme–inducing AEDs such as phenytoin, barbiturates, and carbamazepine lower tiagabine plasma concentrations.
- No significant effect on plasma concentration of other AEDs.
- No significant interaction with oral contraceptives.
- No significant protein-binding interactions.

Elimination

- Eliminated by hepatic metabolism with first-order kinetics
- No active metabolites

Daily Dose

- Adults: up to 52 mg
- Children: not well established
- Daily dose administered in two to three divided doses

Efficacy

- Partial seizures with or without secondary generalization
- Adjunctive therapy

Principal Adverse Effects

- Dose-related: dizziness, headaches, cognitive slowing, drowsiness, nausea, fatigue
- Idiosyncratic/allergic: rare
- Chronic: no reports of serious systemic toxicity
- Teratogenicity: unknown

Advantages

- Well tolerated by majority of patients
- Serum levels not required
- No significant interaction with oral contraceptives
- No reports of serious systemic toxicity

Disadvantages

- Short half-life
- Drug interactions with hepatic enzyme-inducing AEDs
- No parenteral formulation
- Relatively more expensive than traditional AEDs
- Teratogenicity unknown

Topiramate (Topamax)

Chemical Features

- Derived from fructose; contains a sulfamate group
- Poorly water soluble

Mechanism of Action

- Use-dependent sodium channel blocker
- Enhances GABA-mediated transmission
- Inhibitory effect on AMPA glutamate receptors
- Weak carbonic anhydrase inhibitory activity probably does not contribute to its antiepileptic properties

Pharmacology

- Absorption
  - Complete and rapid absorption.
  - Time to reach peak plasma concentration is 1–4 hours.
  - Not altered by administration with meals.
- Protein binding: minimal, 10–15%
- Half-life: 12–24 hours
- Therapeutic range: not established

- Drug interactions
  - Plasma concentration reduced by hepatic enzyme-inducing AEDs, such as carbamazepine and phenytoin
  - May increase plasma level of phenytoin
- Elimination: eliminated mainly unchanged by renal excretion; partially metabolized

Daily Dose

- Adults: 200–1,000 mg (usual dose 200–400 mg).
- Initiate therapy with 25 or 50 mg per day.
- Children: 5–9 mg/kg; initiate with 1 mg/kg.

Efficacy

- Adjunctive therapy in the treatment of partial and secondarily generalized seizures.
- Open-label studies have shown efficacy against various types of primary generalized seizures.

Principal Adverse Effects

- Dose-related: dizziness, headache, drowsiness, tremor, ataxia, fatigue, cognitive difficulties, paresthesias, gastrointestinal upset
- Idiosyncratic/allergic: Psychosis reported but rare
- Chronic
  - Weight loss in 10% of patients, may be severe
  - Nephrolithiasis in 1.5% of patients
- Teratogenicity
  - None reported
  - Teratogenic potential unknown

Advantages

- High efficacy
- Relatively broad spectrum
- Few drug interactions
- Favorable pharmacokinetics
- No enzyme induction of other AEDs
- Twice-daily dosing
- Serum levels not required

Disadvantages

- Relatively high incidence of cognitive and other neurotoxicity

- Kidney stones (rare)
- Possible teratogenicity based on preclinical testing
- Relatively expensive compared with traditional AEDs
- Induction of oral contraceptive hormones

Valproate (Depakote, Epival in Canada, Depakene Syrup, Depacon IV, Epiject IV in Canada)

Chemical Features

- Marketed in North America as acid form or as sodium salt
- 2-*N*-Propylpentanoic acid, a branched-chain amino acid
- Highly water soluble

Mechanism of Action

- Mechanism of action is unclear, likely multiple
- Inhibitory effect on thalamocortical circuit
- Enhances GABA-ergic function in substantia nigra
- Reduces sustained repetitive firing
- May influence sodium and calcium channels

Pharmacology

- Absorption
  - Rapid and complete absorption.
  - Peak plasma concentration reached in 0.5–2.0 hours.
  - With slow-release formulation, peak plasma concentration reached in 3–7 hours.
  - Food delays rate, but not extent, of absorption.
- Protein binding
  - Highly protein bound, saturable (i.e., diminishes at higher serum levels): approximately 90%
  - Susceptible to protein-binding interactions
  - Decreased protein binding during pregnancy and in presence of renal or hepatic disease and other hypoalbuminemic states
- Half-life
  - 6–18 hours, mean 8–9 hours
  - Longer in neonates, shorter in children
  - Shorter in polytherapy
  - Longer in presence of hepatic disease
- Therapeutic range
  - Poorly defined.
  - 50–100 μg/ml (350–700 μmol/liter) are the usual levels achieved with therapeutic doses.

- Drug interactions
  - Increases plasma phenobarbital concentration.
  - May increase concentration of carbamazepine 10,11-epoxide.
  - Interaction with phenytoin complex; has variable effect on the total plasma concentration but may increase free fraction of phenytoin.
  - Phenytoin, carbamazepine, phenobarbital, and primidone stimulate valproate metabolism.
  - May displace diazepam from protein-binding sites.
  - Inhibits lamotrigine metabolism.
  - Salicylates increase free fraction of valproate.
  - Adverse pharmacodynamic interaction between valproate and clonazepam may result in absence status.
  - Valproate does not reduce efficacy of oral contraceptives.
- Elimination
  - Elimination by hepatic metabolism with first-order kinetics.
  - Polytherapy with hepatic enzyme-inducing AEDs increases clearance.
  - Clearance in children is higher than in adults.
  - Clearance increases during pregnancy.
  - Elimination may be reduced in the presence of significant hepatic disease.

Daily Dose

- Adults: 1,000–2,500 mg.
- Children: 15–60 mg/kg.
- Initiate therapy in children at 10–15 mg/kg per day in two or three divided doses.
- Higher doses required when valproate used in polytherapy with other hepatic enzyme inducers.

Efficacy

- Primary generalized seizures: tonic-clonic, absence, myoclonic, tonic, atonic
- Partial seizures

Principal Adverse Effects

- Dose-related: fatigue, tremor, behavioral changes, encephalopathy with stupor or coma, alopecia, hyperammonemia, gastrointestinal upset.
- Idiosyncratic/allergic: bone marrow suppression, hepatotoxicity, pancreatitis, rare skin rash. Although mild thrombocytopenia and mild elevations of liver enzymes are common, serious hepatic toxicity is rare. In children younger than 2 years of age on polytherapy (high-risk group), the incidence of fatal hepatic dysfunction is approximately 1 in 500. This risk declines with age, and in adults on valproate monotherapy the risk is approximately 1 in 45,000.

- Chronic
  - Weight gain
  - Polycystic ovaries, menstrual irregularities, hyperandrogenism
  - Rare reports of encephalopathy and reversible brain atrophy
- Teratogenicity
  - Congenital anomalies reported with other AEDs are also reported with valproate.
  - Risk of spina bifida with exposure in the first trimester is 1–2%.

Advantages

- Broad spectrum
- Rare idiosyncratic reactions (e.g., skin rash)
- Few long-term tissue or cognitive effects
- No hepatic enzyme induction (no interaction with oral contraceptives)
- Mood stabilizer
- Headache prophylaxis in patients with concurrent migraine
- Parenteral preparation available
- Syrup (Depakene), IV, and sprinkle preparation available

Disadvantages

- Weight gain common
- Rare severe hepatotoxicity or pancreatitis
- Teratogenicity (spina bifida in 1–2%)
- Occasional persistent gastrointestinal upset
- Polycystic ovaries, hyperandrogenism, occasional menstrual irregularities
- Drug interactions

Vigabatrin (Sabril)

Chemical Features

- A structural analog of GABA
- Highly water soluble
- Exists as racemic form

Mechanism of Action

- Irreversible inhibition of GABA transaminase, the major degrading enzyme of GABA
- Increases GABA concentration in the brain by 300%
- Activity related to S(+) enantiomer

Pharmacology

- Absorption
  - Well absorbed: 80%.
  - Time to peak concentration is 2 hours.
  - Administration with food does not alter bioavailability.
- Protein binding
  - No protein binding
  - No protein-binding interactions
- Half-life
  - 5–8 hours (probably irrelevant to clinical effect).
  - Increased in older patients and in presence of renal disease.
  - Half-life of GABA-transaminase inhibition is 4–5 days.
- Therapeutic range: no correlation between plasma level and therapeutic effect
- Drug interactions
  - Minor
  - May cause a mild decrease in phenytoin concentration (up to 2%)
  - No interaction with oral contraceptives
- Elimination
  - Excreted unchanged in the urine
  - Correlates with creatinine clearance

Daily Dose

- Adults: 2,000–4,000 mg.
- Children: 80–100 mg/kg.
- Adults: Initiate therapy with 500–1000 mg daily and increase by 500-mg increments.
- Children: Initiate therapy at 40 mg/kg daily.
- Can be given in twice-daily dosing.

Efficacy

- Adjunctive therapy in partial seizures with or without secondary generalization.
- Infantile spasms.
- Monotherapy can be achieved in some patients.

Principal Adverse Effects

- Dose-related: fatigue, drowsiness, behavioral changes, headache, ataxia, gastrointestinal upset
- Idiosyncratic/allergic
  - Rare allergic reactions.

  - Psychosis or severe depression (in 2–4%), usually in the first few months of therapy and preceded by a prodrome of behavioral change such as withdrawal, suspiciousness, or irritability; reversible with discontinuation. Requires close observation and hospitalization in severe cases. Patients and families should be warned to report behavior changes immediately.
- Chronic
  - Weight gain.
  - May aggravate primary generalized seizures (especially absences).
  - No cognitive side effects.
  - *Retinal toxicity* with long-term use causing peripheral concentric field constriction and, in rare cases, symptomatic tunnel vision. Incidence is not yet known, but it appears to be approximately 20% (vast majority asymptomatic). Effect is not dose related; it appears to be permanent. Detected earliest on static 60-degree perimetry (Humphrey's perimeter). Electroretinography (ERG) may be abnormal; visual acuity is normal; visual evoked potentials are normal. Screening with formal visual fields, eye examination, and confrontation fields is recommended before starting the drug and every 3 months in symptomatic patients; the same tests should be performed on asymptomatic patients every 6 months. Visual fields cannot be reliably tested before patients are 10 years of age.
- Teratogenicity
  - None reported
  - Teratogenic potential unknown

Advantages

- Well tolerated
- No long-term cognitive side effects
- Minimal drug interactions
- Twice- or once-daily dosing
- No enzyme induction
- Favorable pharmacokinetics
- Serum levels not required
- High efficacy
- Useful in infantile spasms
- Appears effective in monotherapy
- Potential low teratogenicity

Disadvantages

- Peripheral retinal degeneration with visual field constriction; requires monitoring
- Psychosis or severe depression in 2–4%
- May worsen absence and myoclonic seizures

- Relatively expensive compared with traditional AEDs
- No parenteral form

Suggested Reading

Individual Antiepileptic Drugs

Anhut H, Ashman P, Feverskin TJ, et al. Gabapentin (neurontin) as add-on therapy in patients with partial seizures: a double-blind, placebo-controlled study. Epilepsia 1994;35: 795-801.

Ben-Menachem E. International experience with tiagabine add-on therapy. Epilepsia 1995; 36(Suppl 6):S14-S21.

Ben-Menachem E. Vigabatrin. Epilepsia 1996;36(Suppl 2):S95-S104.

Bergey GK, Morris HH, Rosenfeld W, et al. Gabapentin monotherapy part I: an 8-day, double-blind, dose-controlled, multicenter study in hospitalized patients with refractory complex partial or secondarily generalized seizures. Neurology 1997;49:739-745.

Besag FMC, Wallace SJ, Dulac O, et al. Lamotrigine for the treatment of epilepsy in childhood. J Pediatr 1995;127:991-997.

Beydoun A, Fischer J, Labar DR, et al. Gabapentin monotherapy part II: a 26-week, double-blind, dose-controlled multicenter study of conversion from polytherapy in outpatients with refractory complex partial or secondarily generalized seizures. Neurology 1997;49:746-752.

Boas J, Dam M, Friis ML, et al. Controlled trial of lamotrigine for treatment-resistant partial seizures. Acta Neurol Scand 1996;94:247-252.

Bourgeois B. Felbamate. Semin Pediatr Neurol 1997;4:3-8.

Bourgeois B, Leppik IE, Sackellares JC, et al. Felbamate: a double-blind controlled trial in patients undergoing presurgical evaluation of partial seizures. Neurology 1993;43: 693-696.

Brodie MJ. Lamotrigine—an update. Can J Neurol Sci 1996;23(Suppl 2):S6-S9.

Brodie MJ, Dichter MA. Antiepileptic drugs. N Engl J Med 1996;334:168-175.

Brodie MJ, Pellock JM. Taming the brainstorms: felbamate updated. Lancet 1995;346: 918-919.

Brodie MJ, Richens A, Yuen AWC, et al. Double-blind comparison of lamotrigine and carbamazepine in newly-diagnosed epilepsy. Lancet 1995;345:476-479.

Brodie MJ, Yuen AWC. Lamotrigine substitution study: evidence for synergism with sodium valproate? Epilepsy Res 1997;26:423-432.

Browne TR, Mattson RH, Penry JK, et al. Vigabatrin for refractory complex partial seizures: a multicenter single-blind study with long-term follow-up. Neurology 1987;37:184-189.

Bruni J. Gabapentin. Can J Neurol Sci 1996;23(Suppl 2):S10-S12.

Bruni J. Titration of gabapentin dose for optimal control of epileptic seizures. Adv Therapeutics 1996;13:324-333.

Bruni J. Outcome evaluation of gabapentin as add-on therapy for partial seizures. Can J Neurol Sci 1998;25:134-140.

Chadwick DW, Marson I, Kadir Z. Clinical administration of new antiepileptic drugs: an overview of safety and efficacy. Epilepsia 1996;37(Suppl 6):S17-S22.

Chiron C, Dumas C, Jambaque I, et al. Randomized trial comparing vigabatrin and hydrocortisone in infantile spasms due to tuberous sclerosis. Epilepsy Res 1997;26:389-395.

Christie W, Krämer G, Vigonius V, et al. A double-blind controlled clinical trial: oxcarbazepine versus sodium valproate in adults with newly diagnosed epilepsy. Epilepsy Res 1997;3:451-460.

Dam M, Ekberg R, Loyning Y, et al. A double-blind study comparing oxcarbazepine and carbamazepine in patients with newly diagnosed, previously untreated epilepsy. Epilepsy Res 1989;3:70-76.

Dam M, Ostergaard LH. Other Antiepileptic Drugs: Oxcarbazepine. In RH Levy, RH Mattson, BS Meldrum, et al. (eds), Antiepileptic Drugs (4th ed). New York: Raven, 1995; 987-995.

De Silva M, MacArdle B, McGowan M, et al. Randomized comparative monotherapy trial of phenobarbitone, phenytoin, carbamazepine, or sodium valproate for newly-diagnosed childhood epilepsy. Lancet 1996;347:709-713.

Dichter MA, Brodie MJ. New antiepileptic drugs. N Engl J Med 1996;334:1583-1590.

Dodrill CB, Arnett JL, Sommerville KW, et al. Cognitive and quality of life effects of differing dosages of tiagabine in epilepsy. Neurology 1997;48:1025-1031.

Donaldson JA, Glauser TA, Olberding LS. Lamotrigine adjunctive therapy in childhood epileptic encephalopathy (the Lennox-Gastaut syndrome). Epilepsia 1997;38:68-73.

Eriksson A-S, Nergardh A, Hoppu K. The efficacy of lamotrigine in children and adolescents with refractory generalized epilepsy: a randomized, double-blind, crossover study. Epilepsia 1998;39:495-501.

Faught E, Wilder BJ, Ramsay RE, et al. Topiramate placebo-controlled dose-ranging trial in refractory partial epilepsy using 200-, 400-, and 600-mg daily dosages. Topiramate YD Study Group. Neurology 1996;46:1684-1690.

Felbamate Study Group in the Lennox-Gastaut Syndrome. Efficacy of felbamate in childhood epileptic encephalopathy (Lennox-Gastaut syndrome). N Engl J Med 1993;328:29-33.

Fisher R, Blum D. Clobazam, oxcarbazepine, tiagabine, topiramate, and other new antiepileptic drugs. Epilepsia 1995;36(Suppl 2):S105-S114.

Fisher R, Kälviäinen R, Tanganelli P, et al. Newer antiepileptic drugs as monotherapy: data on vigabatrin. Neurology 1996;47(Suppl 1):S2-S5.

Fitton A, Goa KL. Lamotrigine: an update of its pharmacology and therapeutic uses. Drugs 1995;50:691-713.

French JA, Mosier M, Walker S, et al. A double-blind, placebo-controlled study of vigabatrin three g/day in patients with uncontrolled complex partial seizures. Neurology 1996;46:54-61.

Giardina WJ. Anti-convulsant action of tiagabine, a new GABA-uptake inhibitor. J Epilepsy 1994;7:161-166.

Gilliam F, Vazquez B, Sackellares JC, et al. An active-control trial of lamotrigine monotherapy for partial seizures, Neurology 1998;51:1018-1025.

Glantz MJ, Cole BF, Friedberg MH, et al. A randomized, blinded, placebo-controlled trial of divalproex sodium prophylaxis in adults with newly diagnosed brain tumors. Neurology 1996;46:985-991.

Grant SM, Faulds D. Oxcarbazepine. A review of its pharmacology and therapeutic potential in epilepsy, trigeminal neuralgia and affective disorders. Drugs 1992;43:873-888.

Guberman A. Vigabatrin. Can J Neurol Sci 1996;23(Suppl 2):S13-S17.

Harden CL. New antiepileptic drugs. Neurology 1994;44:787-795.

Heller AJ, Chesterman P, Elwes RDC, et al. Phenobarbitone, phenytoin, carbamazepine or sodium valproate for newly diagnosed adult epilepsy: a randomized comparative monotherapy trial. J Neurol Neurosurg Psychiatry 1995;58:44-50.

Jawad S, Richens A, Goodwin G, et al. Controlled trial of lamotrigine for refractory seizures. Epilepsia 1989;30:356-363.

Jensen PK. Felbamate in the treatment of refractory partial onset seizures. Epilepsia 1993;34(Suppl 7):S25-S29.

Kälviäinen R, Aikiä M, Mervaala E, et al. Long-term cognitive and EEG effects of tiagabine in drug-resistant partial epilepsy. Epilepsy Res 1996;25:291-297.

Kälviäinen R, Aikiä M, Saukkonen A, et al. Vigabatrin versus carbamazepine monotherapy in patients newly diagnosed with epilepsy: a randomized controlled study. Arch Neurol 1995;42:989-996.

Leach JP, Brodie MJ. New antiepileptic drugs—an explosion of activity. Seizure 1995;4:5-17.

Leppik IE, Dreifuss FE, Pledger GW, et al. Felbamate for partial seizures: results of a controlled clinical trial. Neurology 1991;41:1785-1789.

Leppik IE, Graves N, Devinsky O. New antiepileptic medications. Neurol Clin 1996;11: 923-950.

Levy RH (ed). Recent advances in antiepileptic drug pharmacokinetics. Epilepsia 1995;36(Suppl 5):S1-S29.

Levy RH, Mattson RH, Meldrum BS (eds). Antiepileptic Drugs (4th ed). New York: Raven, 1995.

Mackay FJ, Wilton LV, Pearce GL, et al. Safety of long-term lamotrigine in epilepsy. Epilepsia 1997;38:881-886.

Marson AG, Kadir ZA, Chadwick DW. New antiepileptic drugs: a systematic review of their efficacy and tolerability. BMJ 1996;313:1169-1174.

Matsuo F, Bergen D, Faught E, et al. Placebo-controlled study of the efficacy and safety of lamotrigine in patients with partial seizures. Neurology 1993;43:2284-2291.

Mattson RH. Efficacy and adverse effects of established and new antiepileptic drugs. Epilepsia 1995;36(Suppl 2):S13-S26.

Mattson RH, Cramer JA, Collins JF, et al. Comparison of carbamazepine, phenobarbital, phenytoin and primidone in partial and secondarily generalized tonic-clonic seizures. N Engl J Med 1985;313:145-151.

Mattson RH, Cramer JA, Collins JF, et al. A comparison of valproate with carbamazepine for the treatment of complex partial seizures and secondarily generalized tonic-clonic seizures in adults. N Engl J Med 1992;327:765-771.

McKee PJW, Blacklaw J, Butler E, et al. Monotherapy with conventional and controlled release carbamazepine: a double-blind, double-dummy comparison in epileptic patients. Br J Clin Pharmacol 1991;32:99-104.

McLean MJ. Gabapentin. Epilepsia 1996;36(Suppl 2):S73-S86.

Messenheimer JA. Lamotrigine. Epilepsia 1996;36(Suppl 2):S87-S94.

Messenheimer J, Ramsay RE, Willmore LJ, et al. Lamotrigine therapy for partial seizures: a multicenter placebo-controlled, double-blind, crossover trial. Epilepsia 1994;35:113-121.

Palmer KJ, Tavish D. Felbamate—a review of its pharmacodynamic and pharmacokinetic properties, and therapeutic efficacy in epilepsy. Drugs 1993;45:1041-1065.

Pellock J. Antiepileptic drug therapy in the United States. Neurology 1995;45(Suppl 2): S17-S24.

Privitera MD. Topiramate: a new antiepileptic drug. Ann Pharmacother 1997;31:1164-1173.

Privitera M, Fincham R, Penry J, et al. Topiramate placebo-controlled dose-ranging trial in refractory partial epilepsy using 600-, 800-, and 1000-mg daily dosages. Topiramate YE Study Group. Neurology 1996;46:1678-1683.

Ramsay RE, Pellock JM, Garnett WR, et al. Pharmacokinetics and safety of lamotrigine (Lamictal) in patients with epilepsy. Epilepsy Res 1991;10:191-200.

Reunanen M, Dam M, Yuen AWC. A randomized open multicenter comparative trial of lamotrigine and carbamazepine as monotherapy in patients with newly diagnosed or recurrent epilepsy. Epilepsy Res 1996;23:149-155.

Richens A, Davidson DLW, Cartlidge NEF, et al. on behalf of the Adult EPITEG Collaborative Group. A multicenter comparative trial of sodium valproate and carbamazepine in adult onset epilepsy. J Neurol Neurosurg Psychiatry 1994;57:682-687.

Riefe RA, Pledger GW. Topiramate as adjunctive therapy in refractory partial epilepsy: pooled analysis of data from five double-blind, placebo-controlled trials. Epilepsia 1997;38(Suppl 1):S31-S33.

Robertson MM. Current status of the 1,4 and 1,5 benzodiazepines in the treatment of epilepsy: the place of clobazam. Epilepsia 1986;27(Suppl 1):S27-S41.

Rosenfeld WE, Liao S, Kramer LD, et al. Comparison of the steady-state pharmacokinetics of topiramate and valproate in patients with epilepsy during monotherapy and concomitant therapy. Epilepsia 1997;38:324-333.

Sachdeo R, Kramer LD, Rosenberg A, et al. Felbamate monotherapy: controlled trial in patients with partial onset seizures. Ann Neurol 1992;32:386-392.

Sachdeo RC, Leroy RF, Krausr GL, et al. Tiagabine therapy for complex partial seizures. Arch Neurol 1997;54:595-601.

Sachdeo RC, Reife R, Pilar L, et al. Topiramate monotherapy for partial onset seizures. Epilepsia 1997;38:294-300.

Sachdeo RC, Sachdeo SK, Walker SA, et al. Steady-state pharmacokinetics of topiramate and carbamazepine in patients with epilepsy during monotherapy and concomitant therapy. Epilepsia 1996;37:774-780.

Schacter SC. Tiagabine monotherapy in the treatment of partial epilepsy. Epilepsia 1995; 36(Suppl 6):S2-S6.

Tanganelli P, Regesta G. Vigabatrin versus carbamazepine monotherapy in newly diagnosed focal epilepsy: a randomized response conditional cross-over study. Epilepsy Res 1996; 25:257-262.

Tassinari CA, Michelucci R, Chauvel P, et al. Double-blind, placebo-controlled trial of topiramate (600 mg daily) for the treatment of refractory partial epilepsy. Epilepsia 1996;37: 763-768.

The Canadian Clobazam Study Group for Childhood Epilepsy. Monotherapy clobazam versus carbamazepine versus phenytoin in childhood epilepsy: a double-blind randomized trial with 220 Canadian children. Can J Neurol Sci 1996;23(Suppl 1):S18.

US Gabapentin Study Group No. 5. Gabapentin as add-on therapy in refractory partial epilepsy. Neurology 1993;43:2292-2298.

Verity CM, Hosking G, Easter DJ. A multicenter comparative trial of sodium valproate and carbamazepine in pediatric epilepsy. Dev Med Child Neurol 1995;37:97-108.

Walker MC, Patsalos PN. Clinical pharmacokinetics of new antiepileptic drugs. Pharmacol Ther 1995;67:351-384.

Walker MC, Sander JWAS. The impact of new antiepileptic drugs on the prognosis of epilepsy. Neurology 1996;46:912-914.

Wilder BJ. Antiepileptic drugs—current use. Can J Neurol Sci 1996;23(Suppl 2):S18-S23.

Willmore LJ, Shu V, Wallin B, and the M88-194 Study Group. Efficacy and safety of add-on-divalproex sodium in the treatment of complex partial seizures. Neurology 1996;46: 49-53.

Side Effects of Antiepileptic Drugs

Beghi E, DeMascio R, Sasanelli F, et al. Adverse reactions to antiepileptic drugs: a multicenter survey of clinical practice. Epilepsia 1986;27:323-30.

Berlin CM, et al. Behavorial and cognitive effects of anticonvulsant therapy. Pediatrics 1995;96:538-540.

Bruni J. Antiepileptic drug selection and adverse effects: an overview. Can J Neurol Sci 1994;21(Suppl 3):S3-S6.

Bryant AE, Dreifuss FE. Valproic acid hepatic fatalities (part III). U.S. experience since 1986. Neurology 1996;46:465-469.

Dodrill CB, Troupin AS. Neuropsychological effects of carbamazepine and phenytoin: a reanalysis. Neurology 1991;41:141-143.

Dooley J, Camfield P, Gordon K, et al. Lamotrigine-induced rash in children. Neurology 1996;46:240-242.

Eke T, Talbot JF, Lawden MC. Severe persistent visual field constriction associated with vigabatrin. BMJ 1997;314:180-181.

Gallassi R, Morreale A, Lorusso S, et al. Carbamazepine and phenytoin: comparison of cognitive effects in epileptic patients during monotherapy and withdrawal. Arch Neurol 1988;45:892-894.

Gallassi R, Morreale A, Lorusso S, et al. Cognitive effects of valproate. Epilepsy Res 1990;5:160-164.

Herranz JL, Armjo JA, Arteaga R. Clinical side effects of phenobarbital, primidone, phenytoin, carbamazepine, and valproate during monotherapy in children. Epilepsia 1988;29:794-804.

Isajärvi JIT, Laatikainen TJ, Pakarinen AJ, et al. Polycystic ovaries and hyperandrogenism in women taking valproate for epilepsy. N Engl J Med 1993;329:1383-1388.

Krauss GL, Johnson MA, Miller NR. Vigabatrin—associated retinal cone system dysfunction: electroretinogram and ophthalmologic findings. Neurology 1998;50:614-618.

Leach JP, Girvan J, Paul A, et al. Gabapentin and cognition: a double-blind, dose ranging, placebo controlled study in refractory epilepsy. J Neurol Neurosurg Psychiatry 1997;62:372-376.

Levy RH, Penry JK. Idiosyncratic Reactions to Valproate: Clinical Risk Patterns and Mechanisms of Toxicity. New York: Raven, 1991.

Meador KJ, Loring DW, Allen ME, et al. Comparative cognitive effects of carbamazepine and phenytoin in healthy adults. Neurology 1991;41:1537-1540.

Ney GC, Lambs G, Barr WB, et al. Cerebellar atrophy in patients with long-term phenytoin exposure and epilepsy. Arch Neurol 1994;51:767-771.

Pellock JM. Carbamazepine side effects in children and adults. Epilepsia 1987;28(Suppl 3):S64-S70.

Roujeau JC, Stern RS. Severe adverse cutaneous reactions to drugs. N Engl J Med 1994;331:1272-1285.

Schlienger RG, Knowles SK, Shear NH. Lamotrigine-associated anticonvulsant hypersensivity syndrome. Neurology 1998;51:1172-1175.

Schmidt D. Toxicity of Antiepileptic Drugs. In TA Pedley, BS Meldrum (eds), Recent Advances in Epilepsy 3. Edinburgh: Churchill Livingstone, 1986;211-232.

Schmidt D, Krämer G. The new anticonvulsant drugs: implications for avoidance of adverse effects. Drug Safety 1994;11:422-431.

Smith DB, Mattson RH, Cramer JA, et al. Results of a nation-wide Veterans Administration Cooperative Study comparing the efficacy and toxicity of carbamazepine, phenobarbital, phenytoin and primidone. Epilepsia 1987;28(Suppl 3):S50-S58.

Theodore WH, Porter RJ. Removal of sedative-hypnotic antiepileptic drugs from the regimen of patients with intractable epilepsy. Ann Neurol 1983;13:320-324.

Thompson PJ, Trimble MR. Anticonvulsant drugs and cognitive functions. Epilepsia 1982;23:531-544.

Vermeulen J, Aldenkamp AP. Cognitive side-effects of chronic antiepileptic drug treatment: a review of 15 years of research. Epilepsy Res 1995;22:65-95.

7 Special Management Considerations

Neonatal Seizures

- Seizures that occur in the first 28 days of life.
- Occur in approximately 5 of 1,000 live births.
- Seizures in neonate may be difficult to recognize (subtle seizures).
- May be the only manifestation of CNS dysfunction.
- Etiology varies according to time of onset.
- Clinical manifestations are highly variable and may include clonic movements, tonic posturing, apnea (usually unassociated with bradycardia), myoclonic movements, ocular movements, oral-lingual movements, or more complex movements such as rowing movements of the arms or bicycling movements of the legs.
- May or may not occur in association with EEG changes.

Etiology

- Seizures caused by ischemia, hypoxia, or intracerebral hemorrhage occur in the first 2–3 days of life. Metabolic disturbances such as hypocalcemia, pyridoxine dependency, or hypomagnesemia are potentially treatable causes.
- Infections and metabolic disturbances are the primary causes of seizures in the first and second weeks of life.
- Seizures with later onset may be secondary to cerebral dysgenesis, infections, trauma, metabolic disturbances including pyridoxine deficiency, phenylketonuria, and other inborn errors of metabolism.

Evaluation

- *History*: Obtain Apgar score, description of events of delivery, and family history, including history of any maternal drug use.
- *Examination*: Examine for craniofacial abnormalities, skin eruptions, bulging fontanelle, level of consciousness, respiratory pattern, focal neurologic signs, hypotonia, and decerebrate posturing.
- *CSF examination* and *blood chemistry* are indicated in every neonate with seizures.

- Biochemical studies should include evaluation of glucose, calcium, magnesium, phosphorus, electrolytes, bicarbonate, blood urea nitrogen, bilirubin, and ammonia.
- Evaluate urinary ketones and screen for amino acidurias.
- *CT* scan is most useful diagnostic imaging study.
- *EEG* is useful in diagnosis of neonate suspected of having an underlying seizure disorder.
  - Interictal discharges are not reliable predictors.
  - Most useful data are obtained from the evaluation of electrographic activity during clinical events.

Treatment

- Establish airway; ensure oxygenation and circulation.
- Correct and treat underlying conditions when possible (e.g., electrolyte disturbances, sepsis, hypoglycemia, hypocalcemia).
  - Hypoglycemia—0.25–0.50 g/kg bolus of 10% dextrose followed by 8 mg/kg per minute IV drip prn.
  - Hypocalcemia—10 mg/kg elemental calcium administered slowly via IV as 10% calcium gluconate.
  - Because there is no test for pyridoxine deficiency, administer pyridoxine, 100 mg, for persistent seizures. This test dose should be given during EEG monitoring.
- If seizures persist despite correction of metabolic disturbances or if seizures occur in the absence of a correctable abnormality, AED therapy may be required.
- The AEDs that have been most useful include phenobarbital, phenytoin, and diazepam.
  - Phenobarbital is most frequently used. The phenobarbital loading dose is 15–20 mg/kg IV over 5 minutes. An additional 10–20 mg/kg can be given if necessary.
  - Phenytoin is the second most preferred drug. It may cause cardiac arrhythmias and hypotension and should be given under ECG monitoring. Its loading dose is 20 mg/kg at a rate of 1 mg/kg per minute.
  - The loading dose for diazepam is 0.2–0.3 mg/kg IV; may give up to 0.8 mg/kg per hour through IV injection.
  - Instead of diazepam, lorazepam (0.05–0.10 mg/kg IV) could be substituted.
  - Maintenance therapy with phenobarbital should be considered once the acute seizures are controlled.
- The decision to discontinue maintenance therapy must be individualized.

Prognosis

- Prognosis is determined largely by the underlying cause and the degree of brain injury present.
- Approximately one in three neonates with seizures develops mental retardation or cerebral palsy.

- Mortality is 20–40%.
- Epilepsy may develop later in 30–50% of the infants.
- The prognosis is worse in the presence of neurologic deficits, abnormal interictal EEGs, severe seizures (lasting longer than 1 day), cerebral hypoxia, cerebral malformation, or any combination of these factors.

Seizures in the Elderly

- As the general population ages, the incidence versus age curve for new-onset epilepsy is shifting toward older persons.
- Most epilepsy in older persons is symptomatic, with cerebrovascular disease being the most common cause. Other major causes are neoplasms (primary and secondary), Alzheimer's disease, drug and alcohol toxicity or withdrawal, and CNS infections.
- Epilepsy in older patients often responds well to treatment, but the following special treatment considerations apply:
  - Greater morbidity of uncontrolled seizures (e.g., fractures, cardiovascular stress).
  - Greater susceptibility to cognitive and other neurotoxic side effects of AEDs due to concurrent neurologic illness (e.g., Alzheimer's disease) and possible pharmacodynamic differences with age.
  - Accelerated osteomalacia with phenytoin and carbamazepine.
  - Older patients are at risk of having toxic AED levels because of reduced hepatic metabolism of certain AEDs and reduced clearance of renally excreted drugs.
  - Reduced compliance due to factors such as inability to afford drugs, poor memory, and poor vision.
  - Increased free levels of highly bound drugs, such as phenytoin and valproic acid, caused by reduced protein binding or hypoalbuminemia.
  - Associated medical conditions (e.g., renal, hepatic, or cardiac diseases, malnutrition) affecting drug metabolism or susceptibility to side effects.
  - Greater likelihood of drug interactions because of the larger number of prescription and nonprescription drugs used by older people.
  - Difficulty of distinguishing toxic effects of AEDs from other neurologic symptoms in older patients. Neurotoxic effects may be subtle.
  - Monotherapy with lower doses of the less toxic drugs is ideal.
  - Withdrawal of AEDs should be attempted after a seizure-free period of approximately 2 years if the risk of further seizures is low.

Single Seizures

- Up to 7% of people have a seizure at some time. In many cases, there are specific provoking factors, such as a metabolic derangement or head trauma.
- By definition, epilepsy implies recurrent (i.e., more than one) seizures. However, a patient who has had a single unprovoked seizure and an epileptic

EEG or evidence of a previous cerebral cortical insult or lesion is considered to have a relatively high likelihood of having further seizures; that patient could therefore be diagnosed with epilepsy. Most epileptologists would not treat a patient with a single seizure unless the risk of subsequent seizures was high and there were compelling reasons to minimize the risk of further seizures.

- The literature suggests a recurrence rate of 30–78% after a single unprovoked seizure. Berg and Shinnar, in their 1991 meta-analysis of 16 studies, found a pooled risk of recurrence of 51%.
- In a community-based cohort study conducted by Annegers et al. (1986), just over 50% of patients had a recurrence over a 4-year period. Sixty-one percent of the recurrences were in the first year, and only 7 of 117 recurred after 5 years. The recurrence rate was 77% at 5 years in the group with a remote known cause for their epilepsy compared with 45% in the idiopathic group.
- Other studies have suggested that the following factors tend to predict a higher rate of recurrence:
  - Abnormal neurologic status as judged by neurologic examination or neuroimaging
  - EEG abnormalities (especially epileptiform)
  - Partial seizure
- In 1998, Hauser et al. conducted a prospective study of 204 mostly adult patients with a first unprovoked seizure who were seen within 24 hours. Thirty-three percent recurred over the subsequent 5 years. In those with a recurrence, a third seizure occurred within 5 years in 64% of the idiopathic or cryptogenic group and in 87% of the remote symptomatic group. Two-thirds of the initial seizures were generalized. Seventy-four percent of patients were treated after their first seizure, but up to half of them may have been noncompliant. This study supports the rationale of treating after a second seizure.
- A study by Gilad et al. (1996) demonstrated that AED treatment after an initial unprovoked generalized tonic-clonic seizure in adults significantly lowers the risk of recurrence. Over 3 years, the recurrence rates were 22% in the treated group compared with 71% in the untreated group.
- The multicenter open randomized Italian trial by Musicco et al. (1997) studied first primary or secondarily generalized tonic-clonic seizures in adults (approximately 75% of study group) and children (approximately 25% of study group). It compared recurrence with treatment versus nontreatment over 2 years. Monotherapy with one of the traditional drugs was used in the treated group, and recurrence levels adjusted into the therapeutic range. Twenty-four percent of the treated group and 42% of the nontreated group had recurrences. Fifty-six percent of all recurrences occurred in the first 6 months. The probabilities of achieving a 1- or 2-year remission were 87% and 68%, respectively, in the immediately treated group compared with 83% and 60% in the group receiving delayed treatment. Treatment after a first seizure therefore did not affect the ultimate prognosis for remission.

- Decisions regarding treatment after a single seizure should therefore be made on an individual basis, considering both the negative effects of taking medication and the chances of having a recurrent seizure.

Discontinuing Antiepileptic Drugs

- Discontinuation of AEDs is usually considered once a patient, particularly a child, has been seizure-free for at least 2 years.
- The decision of when and if to discontinue AEDs depends on
  - The estimated risk of recurrence off treatment
  - The potential psychosocial and physical morbidity of recurrent seizures
  - The patient's perception of the adverse effects of continuing AEDs, including physical, psychological, convenience, and cost factors
- Because patients should not drive for a period of 3–6 months after AEDs have been discontinued, many adults elect to remain on AEDs indefinitely. Even so, in younger patients who are seizure-free and who might be exposed to long-term effects of these agents, an attempt should be made to discontinue the drugs despite the possible inconvenience of being unable to drive.
- The American Academy of Neurology published guidelines for AED withdrawal based on an analysis of 53 studies with widely varying etiologies published between 1967 and 1991. Results were as follows:
  - 31.2% of children and 39.4% of adults relapsed.
  - The profile least likely to relapse was seizure-free for 2–5 years on AEDs (mean, 3.5 years), had a normal neurologic examination and IQ, had an EEG that normalized on treatment, and had a single type of seizure: partial or generalized.
- A large, well-controlled Medical Research Council (U.K.) study conducted by Chadwick et al. (1996) followed 1,783 seizure-free (for more than 2 years) adults and children, 40% of whom had partial seizures. Patients were randomized either to the drug withdrawal group or to a group continuing its drugs for the duration of the study. Over 2 years, there was a 41% recurrence rate in the withdrawal group (half of these recurrences occurred during withdrawal) compared with 23% in the nonwithdrawal group. Based on these results, a complicated mathematical formula was proposed, taking into account various prognostic factors, to predict recurrence.
- Four European studies released in 1995 suggested recurrence rates ranging from 23% to 65% after withdrawal.
- The factors that seem to correlate with a higher likelihood of recurrence are older age of onset, certain syndromes such as juvenile myoclonic epilepsy and symptomatic epilepsy, and poor initial control of seizures (i.e., long duration of seizures before achieving control).
- Whether a prewithdrawal EEG predicts recurrence is unclear. EEG abnormalities seem to predict recurrence better in generalized than in partial epilepsy and in pediatric rather than in adult epilepsy. A study by Tinuper et al. (1996) found that in partial epilepsy patients, an epileptiform EEG prewithdrawal did not influence relapse rate, but a worsening EEG *during* with-

drawal did increase the likelihood of relapse. Therefore, an EEG before and during withdrawal may be indicated.

- Subtherapeutic AED serum levels before withdrawal should theoretically lower the likelihood of recurrence, but this possibility has not been studied.
- In patients receiving polytherapy, sedating drugs such as barbiturates or benzodiazepines should be withdrawn first.
- Most drugs should be withdrawn slowly over a period of months, particularly barbiturates and benzodiazepines, which are most likely to lead to withdrawal seizures. If necessary, other drugs can be withdrawn over a period of 6 weeks or less.
- In 1996, Chadwick et al. studied the prognosis for patients who experienced a recurrent seizure after AED withdrawal. The best predictors of subsequent seizures were the previous seizure-free interval (less recurrence with longer interval), having partial seizures at recurrence, and having previously experienced seizures during treatment. Having a seizure after AED withdrawal did not adversely affect long-term prognosis compared to patients who remained on medication and had a recurrent seizure after a long seizure-free interval.

Epilepsy and Pregnancy

Fertility and Hormonal Influences

- Up to 0.5% of pregnancies occur in epileptic women. The number of pregnant women with epilepsy has risen as seizures have been better controlled with modern pharmacotherapy and as enlightened attitudes toward epilepsy have allowed more patients to marry or find partners.
- Fertility may be reduced by 20% in epileptic women due to side effects of AEDs (e.g., polycystic ovaries and menstrual irregularities with valproic acid or induction of sex hormone metabolism by hepatic enzyme-inducing agents).
- In a population-based study conducted in Iceland by Olafsson et al. (1998), the number of offspring in an epileptic population of men and women was compared to age- and sex-matched controls. There was no reduction in fertility, except when mental retardation or congenital neurologic impairment was present. This study suggested that fertility may not be reduced by epilepsy or its treatment.
- Libido is reduced in some epileptic patients and may be restored after temporal lobectomy in patients with temporal lobe foci.
- Oral contraceptive failures are increased four to five times in women with epilepsy, due to induction of estrogen metabolism, and to a lesser extent progestin metabolism, by many AEDs.
- Midcycle bleeding signals risk of contraceptive failure but is not an inevitable sign in patients who are at risk of becoming pregnant due to pill failure.
- Oral contraceptives with more than 35 μg of estradiol are recommended for patients on hepatic enzyme-inducing agents. Some patients may require 1½ tablets daily of an oral contraceptive containing 50 μg of ethinyl estradiol.

- Patients on inducing agents must be warned of the risk of oral contraceptive failure and encouraged to use a concurrent second method of birth control.
- Noninducing agents such as valproate, clobazam, vigabatrin, gabapentin, lamotrigine, and tiagabine do not affect sex hormones and may be a better choice in women on oral contraceptives.
- *Catamenial epilepsy*, as defined by Duncan et al. in 1993, refers to cases of epilepsy in which at least 75% of seizures occur between 4 days before and 6 days after menstruation. Hormonal manipulations, premenstrual acetazolamide, and premenstrual clobazam have been used with limited success.

Seizures Appearing in Pregnancy

Seizures may appear de novo in pregnancy for the following reasons:

- Idiopathic epilepsy appearing for the first time in pregnancy (*gestational epilepsy*, which is rare, refers to seizures appearing only during successive pregnancies)
- Cerebrovascular disease (arteriovenous malformation becoming symptomatic, subarachnoid hemorrhage from ruptured aneurysm, cortical venous and sinus thrombosis [usually peri- or postpartum], embolus from amniotic fluid, air or paradoxical embolus from pelvic or leg vein thrombosis)
- Eclampsia (late in pregnancy or peripartum)
- Tumor becoming symptomatic (e.g., meningioma, which can have estrogen receptors)
- Hyponatremia caused by water retention from oxytocin
- IV lidocaine during epidural anesthesia
- Syncope with a seizure (vasodepressor, decreased venous return from pressure on inferior vena cava, varicosities, etc.)
- Psychogenic seizures (especially peripartum)

Outcome of Pregnancy in Epileptic Women

- A 1.5- to 4.0-fold increase in various adverse pregnancy outcomes (e.g., preeclampsia, vaginal bleeding, anemia, hyperemesis gravidarum, placenta previa, and abruptio placentae) exists in most series, but the nature of the risks varies among patient populations. Prematurity, low birth weight, and neonatal asphyxia are also increased two- to fourfold in some series. An increase in perinatal mortality (stillbirth or death in the first week postpartum) is most consistently reported.
- In general, the fetus is protected from the physiologic effects of maternal seizures, but miscarriages can occur with prolonged seizures or status epilepticus. Direct abdominal trauma from a seizure may be harmful to the fetus.
- The factors involved in these adverse outcomes may be socioeconomic or genetic and may be related to seizures or AEDs. There is some evidence that seizures in the first trimester may increase the risk of fetal malformations (Lindhout et al., 1992).

Effect of Pregnancy on Seizures

- In experimental models, estrogen lowers seizure threshold, whereas progesterone elevates seizure threshold and may have an antiepileptic effect.
- Seizure frequency changes in pregnancy are common, unpredictable, and dependent on a number of factors. According to Yerby and Devinsky's 1994 review, studies have shown an increase in seizures in 17-24% of pregnant epileptic women and a decrease in 5-25%.
- When seizures increase during pregnancy, it is usually in the last trimester or peripartum.
- Possible causes of increased seizures are
  - Decreasing AED levels
  - Elevated estrogen levels
  - Water retention
  - Stress, anxiety
  - Sleep deprivation
- AED levels may decrease progressively during pregnancy due to
  - Increased clearance (increased hepatic blood flow and enzyme activity)
  - Poor compliance (fear of teratogenicity)
  - Decreased protein binding (resulting in enhanced metabolism)
  - Decreased absorption (changes in gastric pH and slowed intestinal motility)
  - Increased volume of distribution (increased body water)
- Virtually all older AEDs that are mainly metabolized by the liver show an increased clearance during pregnancy due to an increase in hepatic blood flow and hepatic microsomal enzyme activity.
- Highly bound drugs such as phenytoin and valproic acid show a decreased total level, reflecting a fall in albumin; this decrease is partially compensated for by a 20-100% increase in free fraction, which tends to offset the clinical effects. Serum levels should be obtained at the end of each trimester. Free levels, for highly protein-bound drugs such as valproic acid or phenytoin, give a better indication of whether dose adjustments are needed.

Teratogenicity of Antiepileptic Drugs

Risks of fetal exposure to AEDs fall into four categories: death, malformations, dysmorphism, developmental delay.

- Numerous studies in the past 20-30 years have suggested a two- to threefold increased risk of malformations (major) or anomalies (minor) in fetuses exposed to AEDs. This risk is not large considering there is a baseline risk of malformations for 2-3% of the general population. The overall risk for fetuses exposed to AEDs is therefore 4-9%. A slightly increased risk exists for fetuses in untreated epileptic mothers, suggesting a role for other factors such as genetics, environment, demographics, increased risk for pregnancy complications, and seizures.
- The risk of malformations in offspring of epileptic mothers has declined since the 1960s, possibly due to increased use of drugs with less teratogenic potential (such as carbamazepine), reduced use of polytherapy, and increased folate supplementation.

- All AEDs have some potential risk, which must be balanced against the risk of seizures in both the fetus and the mother if AEDs are discontinued. Seizures during pregnancy have been associated with an increased risk of fetal injury and fetal, neonatal, and infant mortality (Yerby, 1997).
- Maximum risk of exposure is in the first 4 weeks of gestation, at which time mothers may be unaware of the pregnancy.
- The full-blown *fetal anticonvulsant syndrome*, originally called the *fetal hydantoin syndrome*, is rare and has been described with all of the older AEDs. It includes various degrees and combinations of anomalies and malformations such as facial, limb, and digital malformations; cardiac defects; microcephaly; short stature; and mental retardation. It has also been encountered in offspring of untreated epileptic mothers.
- Valproic acid carries a 1–2% risk of producing spina bifida (usually aperta) in exposed fetuses. Craniofacial anomalies, digital anomalies, and possibly radial aplasia have also been associated with valproic acid.
- In 1991, Rosa et al. reported that carbamazepine is associated with a 0.5–1.0% risk of spina bifida. In 1989, Jones et al. described a pattern of craniofacial and limb malformations and developmental delay in a series of offspring whose mothers were on carbamazepine monotherapy during pregnancy. Similarities between this syndrome and fetal hydantoin syndrome were apparent. The 20% incidence of developmental delay in this group goes against clinical experience and suggests ascertainment bias, and the statistical analysis used in the Jones et al. study has been called into question.
- A meta-analysis of five European prospective controlled studies (Samrén et al., 1997) showed that the relative risk for malformations with exposure to either valproate or carbamazepine compared to healthy mother controls was 4.9.
- Risks of spina bifida (Table 7.1) are increased with
  - Family history of or prior child with spina bifida
  - Folate deficiency
  - High doses or fluctuating blood levels during the day
  - Polytherapy

TABLE 7.1 Antenatal Detection of Spina Bifida Aperta

	Sensitivity	*False-Positive Rate*
Fetal ultrasound at 18 wks	≥88%	1.2%
Maternal serum alpha-fetoprotein	75–80%	?
Amniocentesis for alpha-fetoprotein and acetylcholinesterase at 16 wks	97%	0.4%

Conclusion: Amniocentesis necessary after positive ultrasound.
Note: 1% risk of miscarriage with amniocentesis.
Source: NJ Wald, HS Cuckle, JE Haddow, et al. Letter to the Editor. N Engl J Med 1991;324:769–770.

- Phenytoin, barbiturates, and possibly other AEDs are associated with a mildly increased risk of digital and nail hypoplasia (usually remits by age 4), facial and palatal clefts, or cardiac septal defects.
- The new drugs (gabapentin, lamotrigine, topiramate, tiagabine, and vigabatrin) do not appear to be teratogenic, but the limited experience in patients prevents a definitive statement about their safety.
- Possible mechanisms of teratogenicity with AEDs are:
  - Folate deficiency
  - Epoxide or arene oxide intermediates with certain AEDs (may involve epoxide hydrolase deficiency on a genetic basis; may be elevated with inducing agents in polytherapy)
- *Mutagenicity* of phenytoin has been suggested on the basis of anecdotal reports of neuroblastoma and related rare tumors in exposed offspring but is unproven.
- *Hemorrhagic disease of the newborn* can occur due to induction of vitamin K metabolism by inducing AEDs and deficiency of vitamin K–dependent clotting factors. It tends to occur in the first 24 hours postpartum, involves abdominal hemorrhages (e.g., retroperitoneal), and has a 30% mortality.

Recommendations for Management of Epilepsy in Pregnancy

- Issues must be discussed with all epileptic women with childbearing potential.
- Consideration must be given to whether AEDs are needed. Consider simplification of regimen and optimization of dose *before* pregnancy.
- Generally, AEDs that are effective and well tolerated should not be changed. Initial selection of drugs with the least teratogenic potential, such as carbamazepine, clobazam, or possibly one of the newer drugs, is recommended in women who wish to become pregnant.
- Avoid valproic acid and carbamazepine if there is a family history of or previous child with spina bifida.
- Folate, 0.5–1.0 mg per day, should be given to women with childbearing potential who are on AEDs. The dose could be increased to 5 mg per day in patients trying to conceive. Suggestions that folate could exacerbate seizures exist, but this risk is unproven.
- Enforce necessity of good compliance.
- Monitor AED blood levels (especially free levels). Dose adjustments may be necessary if there are significant declines.
- Obtain fetal ultrasound (high resolution) at 16 and 20 weeks; if ultrasound produces suspicion of spina bifida, take amniocentesis for alpha-fetoprotein.
- Give oral vitamin K supplements, 20 mg per day for 4 weeks prepartum (parenteral preparation must be made up into oral solution by a pharmacist if oral vitamin K is not available).
- Fetuses exposed to barbiturates prepartum may have withdrawal symptoms after the first week postpartum.

- Breast-feeding is generally safe. AEDs enter the breast milk in inverse proportion to their protein binding. Sedating drugs, such as the barbiturates, may cause sedation of the newborn.
- Mothers who are having seizures must be taught precautions when taking care of newborns and young children. Examples of such precautions are changing and feeding the baby while sitting on a blanket on the floor and never bathing the baby alone.

Eclampsia

- Eclampsia is defined as one or more seizures in a patient with preeclampsia. Preeclampsia includes recently elevated blood pressure, proteinuria, and elevated liver enzymes.
- Encephalopathy is related to vasoconstriction, cerebral edema, microhemorrhages, and disseminated intravascular coagulation.
- The seizures are generally tonic-clonic.
- Treatment consists of control of hypertension, management of cerebral edema, and control of seizures.
- Conventional AEDs, such as benzodiazepines or phenytoin, have been used as initial therapy. In 1995, however, Lucas et al. found that magnesium sulfate is more effective than phenytoin in preventing seizures in hypertensive patients during labor and should be used initially.
- For eclamptic seizures, magnesium sulfate can be given IV or IM. The IV loading dose is 4 g over 5 minutes followed by an infusion of 1 g per hour for 24 hours. A further 2–4 g can be given if seizures recur. After an initial loading dose of 4 g IV, 5 g can be given IM in each buttock followed by 5 g every 4 hours with monitoring of urine output (>100 ml per hour), respiratory rate (>12 per minute), and deep tendon reflexes (preserved). It should be used cautiously in uremia, in myasthenia gravis, or with concurrent administration of neuromuscular blocking agents.
- Phenytoin, 10 mg/kg, can be given as a loading dose in resistant cases or in cases with status epilepticus. Because of the reduced protein binding, the loading dose is lower than in nonpregnant patients. A second dose of 5 mg/kg can be given 2-6 hours later. Diazepam, 10 mg (one or two doses), can be given for status epilepticus without a depressant effect on the fetus.

Suggested Reading

Neonatal Seizures

Legido A, Clancy RR, Berman PH. Neurologic outcome after electroencephalographically proven neonatal seizures. Pediatrics 1991;88:583–596.

Lombroso CT, Holmes GL. Value of the EEG in neonatal seizures. J Epilepsy 1993;6:39–70.

Maytal J, Novak GP, King KC. Lorazepam in the treatment of refractory neonatal seizures. J Child Neurol 1991;6:319–323.

Mizrahi EM. Neonatal seizures: problems in diagnosis and classification. Epilepsia 1987;28 (Suppl 1):S46-S55.
Mizrahi EM. Treatment of Neonatal Seizures. In J Engel Jr, TA Pedley (eds), Epilepsy: A Comprehensive Textbook. New York: Lippincott-Raven, 1998;1295-1303.
Mizrahi EM, Plouin P, Kellaway P. Neonatal Seizures. In J Engel Jr, TA Pedley (eds), Epilepsy: A Comprehensive Textbook. New York: Lippincott-Raven, 1998;647-663.
Painter MJ, Gaus LM. Neonatal seizures: diagnosis and treatment. J Child Neurol 1991;6: 101-108.
Scher MS, Painter MJ. Controversies concerning neonatal seizures. Pediatr Clin North Am 1993;91:128-134.
Volpe JJ. Neonatal seizures: current concepts and revised classification. Pediatrics 1989;84: 422-428.

Epilepsy in the Elderly

de la Court A, Breteler MMB, Meinardi H, et al. Prevalence of epilepsy in the elderly: the Rotterdam study. Epilepsia 1996;37:141-147.
Ettinger AB, Shinnar S. New-onset seizures in an elderly hospitalized population. Neurology 1993;43:489-492.
Franson KL, Hay DP, Neppe V, et al. Drug-induced seizures in the elderly. Drugs Aging 1995;7:38-48.
Hauser WA. Seizure disorders: the changes with age. Epilepsia 1992;33(Suppl 4):S6-S14.
Hesdorffer DC, Hauser WA, Annegers JF, et al. Dementia and adult onset unprovoked seizures. Neurology 1996;46:727-730.
Loiseau J, Loiseau P, Duche B, et al. A survey of epileptic disorders in southwest France: seizures in elderly patients. Neurology 1990;27:232-237.
Luhdorf K, Jensen LK, Plesner AM. Etiology of seizures in the elderly. Epilepsia 1986;27: 458-463.
McAreavey MJ, Ballinger BR, Fenton GW. Epileptic seizures in elderly patients with dementia. Epilepsia 1992;33:657-660.
Rowan AJ, Ramsay RE (eds). Seizures and Epilepsy in the Elderly. Boston: Butterworth-Heinemann, 1997.
Scheuer ML. Seizures and Epilepsy in the Elderly. In TA Pedley, BS Meldrum (eds), Recent Advances in Epilepsy (Vol. 6). Edinburgh: Churchill Livingstone, 1995;247-270.
Scheuer ML, Cohen J. Seizures and epilepsy in the elderly. Neurol Clin 1993;11:787-804.
Thomas RJ. Seizures and epilepsy in the elderly. Arch Intern Med 1997;157:605-617.
Willmore LJ. The effect of age on pharmacokinetics of antiepileptic drugs. Epilepsia 1995;36(Suppl 5):S14-S21.

Single Seizures

Annegers JF, Shirts FB, Hauser WA, Kurland LT. Risk of recurrence after an initial unprovoked seizure. Epilepsia 1986;27:43-50.
Berg AT, Shinnar S. The risk of seizure recurrence following a first unprovoked seizure: a quantitative review. Neurology 1991;41:965-972.
Camfield PR, Camfield S, Dooley JM, et al. Epilepsy after a first unprovoked seizure in childhood. Neurology 1985;27:1657-1660.
Chadwick D. Epilepsy after first seizure: risks and implications. J Neurol Neurosurg Psychiatry 1991;54:385-387.

Chadwick D. Prognostic index for recurrence of seizures after remission of epilepsy. BMJ 1993;306:1374-1378.
Elwes RDC, Reynolds EH. The Early Prognosis of Epilepsy. In M Dam, L Gram (eds), Comprehensive Epileptology. New York: Raven, 1991;715-727.
Gilad R, Lampl Y, Gabbay U, et al. Early treatment of a single generalized tonic-clonic seizure to prevent recurrence. Arch Neurol 1996;53:1149-1152.
Hauser WA, Anderson VE, Loewenson RB, et al. Seizure recurrence after a first unprovoked seizure. N Engl J Med 1982;307:522-528.
Hauser WA, Rich SS, Lee JR, et al. Risk of recurrent seizures after 2 unprovoked seizures. N Engl J Med 1998;338:429-434.
Musicco M, Beghi E, Solari A, et al. Treatment of first tonic-clonic seizure does not improve the prognosis of epilepsy. Neurology 1997;49:991-998.
Shinnar S, Berg AT, Moshe SL, et al. The risk of seizure recurrence after a first unprovoked afebrile seizure in childhood: an extended follow-up. Pediatrics 1996;98:216-225.

Discontinuation of Antiepileptic Drugs

Chadwick D, Taylor J, Johnson T, for the MRC Antiepileptic Drug Withdrawal Group. Outcomes after seizure recurrence in people with well-controlled epilepsy and the factors that influence it. Epilepsia 1996;37:1043-1050.
Dooley J, Gordon K, Camfield P, et al. Discontinuation of anticonvulsant therapy in children free of seizures for 1 year. Neurology 1996;46:969-974.
Duncan JS, Shorvon SD, Trimble MR. Withdrawal symptoms from phenytoin, carbamazepine and sodium valproate. J Neurol Neurosurg Psychiatry 1988;51:924-928.
Duncan JS, Shorvon SD, Trimble MR. Discontinuation of phenytoin, carbamazepine and sodium valproate in patients with active epilepsy. Epilepsia 1990;31:324-333.
Medical Research Council of Antiepileptic Drug Withdrawal Study Group. Randomised study of antiepileptic drug withdrawal in patients in remission. Lancet 1991;337:1175-1180.
Overweg J. Withdrawal of antiepileptic drugs in seizure-free patients, risk factors for relapse with special attention to the EEG. Seizure 1995;4:19-36.
Overweg J, Binnie CD, Oosting J, et al. Clinical and EEG prediction of seizure recurrence following antiepileptic drug withdrawal. Epilepsy Res 1987;1:272-283.
Shinnar S, Vining EPG, Mellits ED, et al. Discontinuing antiepileptic medication in children with epilepsy after two years without seizures. N Engl J Med 1985;313:976-980.
Sugai K. Seizures with clonazepam: discontinuation and suggestions for safe discontinuation rates in children. Epilepsia 1993;34:1089-1097.
Tennison M, Greenwood R, Lewis D, et al. Discontinuing antiepileptic drugs in children with epilepsy: a comparison of six-week and nine-month taper period. N Engl J Med 1994;330:1407-1410.
Tinuper P, Avoni P, Riva R, et al. The prognostic value of the electroencephalogram in antiepileptic drug withdrawal in partial epilepsies. Neurology 1996;47:76-78.

Pregnancy and Epilepsy

Annegers JF, Baumgartner KB, Hauser WA, et al. Epilepsy, antiepileptic drugs and the risk of spontaneous abortion. Epilepsia 1988;29:451-458.
Bernus I, Hooper WD, Dickinson RG, et al. Metabolism of carbamazepine and co-administered anticonvulsants during pregnancy. Epilepsy Res 1995;21:65-75.

Bjerkdal T, Bahna SL. The course and outcome of pregnancy in women with epilepsy. Acta Obstet Gynecol Scand 1973;52:245-248.
Buehler BA, Rao V, Finnell RH. Biochemical and molecular teratology of fetal hydantoin syndrome. Neurol Clin 1994;12:741-748.
Cornellison M, Steegers-Theunissen R, Kollee L, et al. Supplementation of vitamin K in pregnant women receiving anticonvulsant therapy prevents neonatal vitamin K deficiency. Am J Obstet Gynecol 1993;168:884-888.
Dansky LV, Andermann E, Rosenblatt D, et al. Anticonvulsants, folate levels and pregnancy outcome: a prospective study. Ann Neurol 1987;21:176-182.
Delgado-Escueta AV, Janz D, Beck-Mannagetta G (eds). Pregnancy and teratogenesis in epilepsy. Neurology 1992;42(Suppl 5):1-160.
Duley L, et al. for the Eclampsia Trial Collaborative Group. Which anticonvulsant for women with eclampsia? Evidence from the Collaborative Eclampsia Trial. Lancet 1995;345:1455-1463.
Duncan S, Read CL, Brodie MJ. How common is catamenial epilepsy? Epilepsia 1993;34: 827-831.
Janz D. Antiepileptic drugs and pregnancy: altered utilization patterns and teratogenesis. Epilepsia 1982;23(Suppl 1):S53-S62.
Janz D, Bossi L, Dam M, et al. (eds). Epilepsy, Pregnancy and the Child. New York: Raven, 1982.
Jones KL, Lacro RV, Johnson KA, et al. Pattern of malformations in the children of women treated with carbamazepine during pregnancy. N Engl J Med 1989;320:1661-1666.
Levy RH, Yerby MS. Effects of pregnancy on antiepileptic drug utilization. Epilepsia 1985;26(Suppl 1):525-557.
Lindhout D, Meinardi H, Meijer WA, et al. Antiepileptic drugs and teratogenesis in two consecutive cohorts: changes in prescription policy paralleled by changes in pattern of malformations. Neurology 1992;42(Suppl 5):94-110.
Lucas MJ, Leveno KJ, Cunningham FG. A comparison of magnesium sulfate with phenytoin for the prevention of eclampsia. N Engl J Med 1995;33:201-205.
Morrell MJ. Hormones and epilepsy through the lifetime. Epilepsia 1992;33(Suppl 4): S49-S61.
Morrell MJ. The new antiepileptic drugs and women: efficacy, reproductive health, pregnancy and fetal outcome. Epilepsia 1996;37(Suppl 6):S34-S44.
Mountain KR, Hirsh J, Gallus AS. Maternal coagulation defect due to anticonvulsant treatment in pregnancy. Lancet 1970;1:265-268.
Nelson KB, Ellenberg JH. Maternal seizure disorder, outcome of pregnancy and neurologic abnormalities in the children. Neurology 1982;32:1247-1254.
Olafsson E, Hauser A, Gudmundsson G. Fertility in patients with epilepsy. A population-based study. Neurology 1998;51:71-73.
Rosa FW. Spina bifida in infants of women treated with carbamazepine during pregnancy. N Engl J Med 1991;324:674-677.
Samrén EB, Van Duijn CM, Kochs, et al. Maternal use of antiepileptic drugs and the risk of major congenital malformations: a joint European prospective study of human teratogenesis associated with maternal epilepsy. Epilepsia 1997;38:981-990.
Yerby MS. Pregnancy and epilepsy. Epilepsia 1991;32(Suppl 6):S51-S59.
Yerby MS. Pregnancy, teratogenesis, and epilepsy. Neurol Clin 1994;12:749-771.
Yerby MS. Teratogenic effects of antiepileptic drugs: what do we advise patients? Epilepsia 1997;38:957-958.
Yerby MS, Devinsky O. Epilepsy and Pregnancy. In O Devinsky, E Feldmann, B Hainline (eds), Neurological Complications of Pregnancy. New York: Raven, 1994;45-63.

Yerby MS, Friel PN, McCormick KB, et al. Pharmacokinetics of anticonvulsants in pregnancy: alterations in plasma protein binding. Epilepsy Res 1990;5:223-228.
Yerby MS, Koepsell T, Daling J. Pregnancy complications and outcomes in a cohort of women with epilepsy. Epilepsia 1985;26:631-635.
Zahn CA, Morrell MJ, Collins SD, et al. Management issues for women with epilepsy. A review of the literature. Neurology 1998;51:949-956.

8 Status Epilepticus

Status epilepticus (SE): A series of closely spaced seizures or a continuous seizure lasting more than 30 minutes. In the case of generalized tonic-clonic seizures, two or more seizures in a row without regaining consciousness.

Epidemiology

- The estimated annual incidence of SE from a 1996 prospective, community-based U.S. study conducted by DeLorenzo et al. is 41-61 per 100,000 persons.
- As with epilepsy in general, the incidence is highest in the first year of life and in persons older than age 65 (Walker, 1998).
- Twelve percent to 30% of adult patients with a new diagnosis of epilepsy present with SE (Lowenstein and Alldredge, 1998).
- Twenty-five percent to 50% of SE occurs in patients with preexisting epilepsy.
- Approximately 15% of patients with epilepsy will have SE at some point.
- Ten percent to 20% of children with epilepsy will have at least one episode of SE (Shinnar et al., 1997).
- Nine percent of children with a first unprovoked seizure presented with SE (Shinnar et al., 1997).
- Children younger than 2 years with SE tended to be otherwise neurologically normal and without previous seizures (Shinnar et al., 1997).
- Novak et al. (1997) identified four factors as increasing the risk of SE in children with symptomatic epilepsy: focal background abnormalities on EEG, history of partial seizures with secondary generalization, generalized abnormalities on neuroimaging, and first seizure as SE.

Classification

- A classification of status is shown in Table 8.1.
- Virtually any seizure type can occur as SE, but some rarely do (e.g., tonic status).

Myoclonic Status

Myoclonic status is most often seen post-cardiac arrest and is indicative of severe anoxic-ischemic brain damage.

TABLE 8.1 Classification of Status Epilepticus

Convulsive
Generalized
 Tonic-clonic
 Other (clonic, myoclonic, tonic)
Partial
 Simple partial motor
 Epilepsy partialis continua
Nonconvulsive
Generalized (absence status)
Partial
 Complex partial
 Simple partial sensory

Epilepsy Partialis Continua

- *Epilepsy partialis continua* is simple partial motor status that consists of repetitive clonic movements (usually of a limb) that continue for days, weeks, months, or years.
- Etiologies include Rasmussen's and other forms of encephalitis, infarcts, tumors, and Alpers' syndrome.
- EEG may or may not show contralateral frontocentral spikes.
- Resistant to treatment.

Nonconvulsive Generalized Status

- *Nonconvulsive generalized status* (also called *absence status, spike-wave stupor*) presents as a confusional state, usually with relatively preserved level of consciousness although stupor may be seen. The EEG shows continuous spike-waves or poly-spike waves bilaterally and synchronously with an anterior predominance. The pattern is irregular and may have interspersed slow waves. It varies in form from patient to patient. It can be confused with triphasic waves accompanying metabolic encephalopathy.
- May occur de novo even in older patients or in the context of known epilepsy.
- Many cases may be secondarily generalized despite the lack of focal EEG findings. Rare in patients with primary generalized epilepsy.
- May be provoked by drugs or drug withdrawal (particularly withdrawal of such drugs as benzodiazepines, tricyclic antidepressants, and phenothiazines).
- Often mistaken for psychiatric conditions such as acute depression and acute catatonic states.
- May have subtle motor manifestations such as intermittent rhythmic eye blinks, brow or facial twitching, or multifocal myoclonic movements.

- Patients may be capable of talking, walking, and feeding themselves, but they often appear confused, with an increased latency of response. Manifestations may be subtle, and EEG confirmation is necessary for diagnosis.
- The episode may consist of a continuous, prolonged seizure with a fluctuating spike-wave appearance on the EEG, or it may consist of discrete, closely spaced absence seizures (often atypical absences) with return to normal EEG and responsiveness for several seconds between seizures.
- The episode may follow an initial generalized tonic-clonic seizure, be punctuated by generalized tonic-clonic seizures, or terminate with a generalized tonic-clonic seizure.
- The status may continue for hours, days, and, rarely, weeks
- Almost all cases respond to IV benzodiazepine, although repeated doses may be necessary. An oral loading dose of clobazam (1 mg/kg) may be effective.
- Many patients have recurrent bouts; valproate is the only chronic treatment that has been shown to prevent recurrence.
- No reported adverse sequelae from this type of status.

Complex Partial Status

- *Complex partial status* consists of closely spaced complex partial seizures with persisting confusion between seizures and "cycling" on the EEG (discrete recurrent ictal activity). It can consist of a more continuous confusional state with or without automatisms and an EEG showing more continuous but fluctuating spike-waves or sharp theta that is more generalized, often with some lateralization or focal predominance.
- Underlying structural brain abnormalities are relatively common.
- Easily misdiagnosed as a psychiatric disorder unless the EEG is done.
- More common with frontal foci than temporal foci; EEG manifestations may be subtle in frontal cases.
- Treatment is more urgent than with nonconvulsive generalized status, because sequelae such as memory deficits and Klüver-Bucy syndrome occur in rare cases.
- Treatment is similar to that for generalized tonic-clonic status, with perhaps less urgency for general anesthesia; an oral clobazam loading dose (1 mg/kg) can be used if initial IV therapy fails (Corman et al., 1998).

Special Forms of Partial Status Epilepticus

- *Aphasic SE*: Temporal lobe status presenting with aphasia as the only feature in a patient who is alert (Grimes et al., 1997).
- *Occipital SE*: Presents as intermittent contralateral eye deviation and nystagmus.
- *Partial motor status with contralateral periodic lateralized epileptiform discharges (PLEDs)* on the EEG: Etiologies include cerebral infarct, hypoxia/ischemia, tumors, herpes simplex encephalitis, abscess, contusion. Not all PLEDs are accompanied by seizures.

Etiology

- Etiologies of SE are shown in Tables 8.2 and 8.3.
- Children younger than 2 years with SE have a high incidence of febrile or acute symptomatic origin. Older children are more likely to have cryptogenic or remote symptomatic causes (Shinnar et al., 1997).
- A large variety of acute brain or systemic metabolic insults can be associated with SE.
- Intoxication by drugs, including tricyclic antidepressants, isonicotinic acid hydrazide (isoniazid), and theophylline, can produce SE.
- Withdrawal from sedatives, hypnotics, narcotics, and AEDs is commonly associated with SE.

Management Principles

- SE must be distinguished from other nonepileptic conditions (Table 8.4).
- Serial seizures that do not involve impairment of consciousness between them should not be called SE, although the dividing line between clusters of seizures (serial seizures) and status is somewhat arbitrary.
- Generalized convulsive SE (GCSE) is a neurologic emergency. Animal studies show that the probability of brain damage and death is higher if the status lasts longer than 60 minutes.
- The electrical seizures must be stopped. Stopping the convulsive movements with paralytic agents and redressing systemic derangements are not enough.
- The significance of GCSE differs in adults and children. There is much greater likelihood of an underlying acute brain abnormality or acute metabolic dis-

TABLE 8.2 Causes* of Status Epilepticus (SE) in 554 Patients from Five Case Series

	SE as Presenting Symptom of Epilepsy (n = 327) (%)	*SE as an Intercurrent Event in Established Epilepsy (n = 227) (%)*
Cerebral trauma	12	17
Cerebral tumor	16	10
Cerebrovascular disease	20	19
Intracranial infection	15	6
Acute metabolic disturbance	12	5
Other acute event	14	3
No cause found	11	41

*Excluding precipitating causes.

Source: Reprinted with permission from S Shorvon. Status Epilepticus. New York: Cambridge University Press, 1994;69.

TABLE 8.3 Etiology of Status Epilepticus in a Community-Based Study

Children	Infections with fever	52%
	Remote symptomatic	39%
	Low antiepileptic blood levels	21%
	Stroke	10%
	Metabolic	7%
	Idiopathic	5%
Adults	Low antiepileptic blood levels	34%
	Remote symptomatic	24%
	Stroke	22%
	Hypoxia	13%
	Metabolic	15%
	Alcohol	13%
	Idiopathic	3%

n = 166; episodes = 204.

Note: Almost 50% of adult cases were due to remote or acute stroke.

Source: RJ DeLorenzo, WA Hauser, AR Towne, et al. A prospective, population-based epidemiologic study of status epilepticus in Richmond, Virginia. Neurology 1996;46:1029–1035.

turbance in adults; mortality is much higher in adults (largely related to the acute concurrent brain disturbances causing status). Febrile seizures in children (especially aged 6 months to 6 years) can present as GCSE.

- Assessment, investigations, and therapy proceed simultaneously.

TABLE 8.4 Differential Diagnosis of Status Epilepticus

Convulsive	*Nonconvulsive*
Adults	Adults
Movement disorders	Pseudoseizure status
Pseudoseizure status	Dissociative states
Tetanus	Fugue states
Malignant hyperthermia	Panic attacks
Malignant neuroleptic syndrome	Hyperventilation/anxiety
Decerebrate spasms	Acute confusional state (metabolic encephalopathy)
Children	Transient global amnesia
Movement disorders	Children
Pseudoseizure status	Pseudoseizure status
Tetanus	Migraine (vertebrobasilar)
Decerebrate spasms	

Management of Generalized Convulsive Status Epilepticus

- First attend to the airway and stabilize vital signs.
- Perform a rapid general and neurologic examination for signs of meningitis, alcohol or drug abuse, raised intracranial pressure, head trauma, and focal neurologic abnormalities.
- Causes (e.g., meningitis, hyponatremia) and precipitants must be searched for and treated.
- In adults, administer 25–50 ml of 50% glucose if hypoglycemia is present or if a glucose determination is not available. Give thiamine, 100 mg IV. Correct electrolyte disturbances, and administer an ampule of bicarbonate for severe acidosis (pH <7.0). In children, give IV 25% glucose, 2 ml/kg.
- If temperature is higher than 39°C, reduce it with cooling blankets.
- Avoid overstimulation through excessive movement or unnecessary suctioning.
- Whether a patient has a known history of epilepsy and was supposed to be taking AEDs does not influence the choice and dose of AEDs used to treat SE (unless the patient is allergic to one of the drugs).
- Drugs should be given IV whenever possible (Table 8.5).
- Benzodiazepines can be given rectally (e.g., outside the hospital); a rectal diazepam gel preparation is available that, according to a 1998 study by Dreifuss et al., has good bioavailability and is effective in acute repetitive seizures and clusters in adults and children.
- Phenobarbital can be given IM in children.
- Fosphenytoin (Cerebyx), a water-soluble prodrug of phenytoin, can be given IM or IV (Ramsay et al., 1997).
  - It is rapidly converted by phosphatases to phenytoin, with a conversion half-life of 15 minutes.
  - The drug is supplied in a ready-mixed solution, pH 9.0, of 50 mg phenytoin equivalents (i.e., 75 mg of fosphenytoin) per ml.
  - It avoids complications of tissue irritation, phlebitis, and rarely necrosis ("purple glove syndrome"), which may be associated with IV phenytoin due to the propylene glycol vehicle. Hypotension is also less.
  - It can be given at three times the IV rate of phenytoin (i.e., 150 mg per minute).
  - It may cause transient paraesthesias or pruritus in the perineal area.
  - Fosphenytoin is much more expensive than phenytoin.
- An IV preparation of valproate is available, but there is limited experience in treating SE with it.

Initial Drug Treatment

- Lorazepam, 2 mg IV (0.05–0.10 mg/kg, up to 4 mg in children), over 2 minutes with additional doses as necessary every 2–3 minutes to a total of 8 mg. Diazepam, 5–10 mg IV (0.3 mg/kg in children), maximum 10 mg, can be substituted, but it has a shorter duration of action because it redistributes to fat

TABLE 8.5 Major Drugs Used to Treat Status Epilepticus: Intravenous Doses, Pharmacokinetics, and Major Toxicities

	Diazepam	*Lorazepam*	*Phenytoin/ Fosphenytoin*	*Phenobarbital*	*Midazolam*	*Thiopental*	*Pentobarbital*	*Propofol*
Adult IV dose, mg/kg (range [total dose])	0.15–0.25 [20–40 mg]	0.1 [4.0–8.0 mg]	20	10–20	0.05–0.30 loading at <4 mg/min (infusion 0.1–0.4 mg/kg/hr); can be given IM	3–4 loading (infusion 50–150 mg/hr)	5–20 loading over 30 mins (infusion 1–4 mg/kg/hr)	2.0–2.5 loading (infusion 6–12 mg/kg/hr); later 1–3 mg/kg/hr
Pediatric IV dose, mg/kg (range [total dose])	0.1–1.0	0.05–0.50 [1–4 mg]	20	10–20 over 15 mins	—	3–5 mg/kg load (infusion 2–4 mg/kg/hr)	5 mg/kg load (infusion 1–3 mg/kg/hr)	—
Pediatric per rectum dose (mg/kg)	0.5 mg/kg (max. 10 mg)	Erratic absorption	—	—	0.15–0.30	—	—	—

TABLE 8.5 *Continued*

	Diazepam	*Lorazepam*	*Phenytoin/ Fosphenytoin*	*Phenobarbital*	*Midazolam*	*Thiopental*	*Pentobarbital*	*Propofol*
Maximal administration rate (mg/min)	5	2.0	50 in adults (150 for fosphenytoin) <3 mg/kg/min in children	100	—	—	25	—
Time to stop status (mins)	1–3	6–10	10–30	20–30	1–3 hrs	—	—	—
Effective duration of action (hrs)	0.25–0.50	>12–24	24	>48	—	—	—	—
Elimination half-life (hrs)	30	14	24	100	1.5–3.5 (10 hrs in older patients)	8–36 days depending on levels	27 days	30–60 mins
Potential side effects								
Depression of consciousness	10–30 mins	Several hours	None	Several days	Minutes	Several days	Days	Hours
Respiratory depression	Occasional	Occasional	Infrequent	Occasional	Occasional	Common	Common	Common
Hypotension	Infrequent	Infrequent	Occasional	Infrequent	Infrequent	Common	Common	Uncommon

Cardiac arrhythmias	—	—	In patients with heart disease	—	—	—	—	Uncommon
Other	—	—	Vein or tissue inflammation (not with fosphenytoin)	—	Long-term infusion may be associated with tachyphylaxis; very expensive	Prolonged coma (accumulates in fat tissue; saturable metabolism)	Involuntary movements; green urine; relatively expensive	—

depots. These doses can be repeated in 15 minutes if seizures recur. Respiratory depression and hypotension must be watched for.

- Phenytoin, 20 mg/kg (or fosphenytoin; see Management of Generalized Convulsive Status Epilepticus), is given IV (as close to the vein as possible to minimize precipitation in the tubing) in normal saline at less than 50 mg per minute in adults and less than 3 mg/kg per minute in children. Lorazepam should be given simultaneously in the opposite arm. Phenytoin may cause local tissue or vein inflammation and, rarely, necrosis. Hypotension or cardiac arrhythmias such as heart block can occur, particularly in older patients. If necessary, a second dose of phenytoin, 10 mg/kg IV, can be given 20 minutes after the first dose is fully infused. Stopping the SE is a more important consideration than acute phenytoin toxicity.
- If seizures continue, phenobarbital, 10 mg/kg IV, repeated once in 10 minutes prn or midazolam (see Table 8.5 for dose) can be used before considering general anesthesia with propofol, thiopental, or pentobarbital.
- By this time, the patient is usually in the ICU and requires intubation for airway protection and possibly ventilatory support. Support of blood pressure with pressor agents may also be necessary. Continued search for underlying causes or precipitants and metabolic or intracranial abnormalities should not be neglected. CT or MRI, and possibly lumbar puncture, should be done in patients in whom etiology is unclear, especially in patients not known to have epilepsy.
- General anesthesia with propofol or barbiturates should be instituted within 60 minutes of onset of resistant status (Figure 8.1). If the patient has had seizures for more than 30 minutes (especially continuous seizures) before arrival at the hospital, the timeline may be compressed, and after an initial trial of a benzodiazepine and phenytoin, general anesthesia may be used within 30 minutes of the onset of treatment.
- The EEG should be monitored whenever possible, especially in resistant status. If a regular EEG is not available, two-channel monitors (available in some ICUs) can be used. Treiman et al. (1990) showed that there is a progression of EEG from continuous epileptic activity to intermittent activity with background slowing, to a burst suppression pattern with progressive background slowing and flattening as status proceeds. When the EEG shows an advanced stage of status with a burst suppression pattern or prolonged background flattening, convulsions may have ceased, giving the false impression that the patient is improving. The stage of SE as revealed by the EEG correlates with the resistance to drug therapy and ultimate outcome.
- With general anesthesia, the objective is to produce a burst suppression pattern on the EEG (approximately one burst every 10 seconds). Burst suppression may be difficult to achieve, however, and may not be necessary as long as electrical epileptic activity is eliminated. After 24 hours, the anesthetic should be tapered and stopped and the EEG recorded to see whether seizure activity is still present. Duration of the anesthesia may be governed by the underlying etiology in addition to the response.

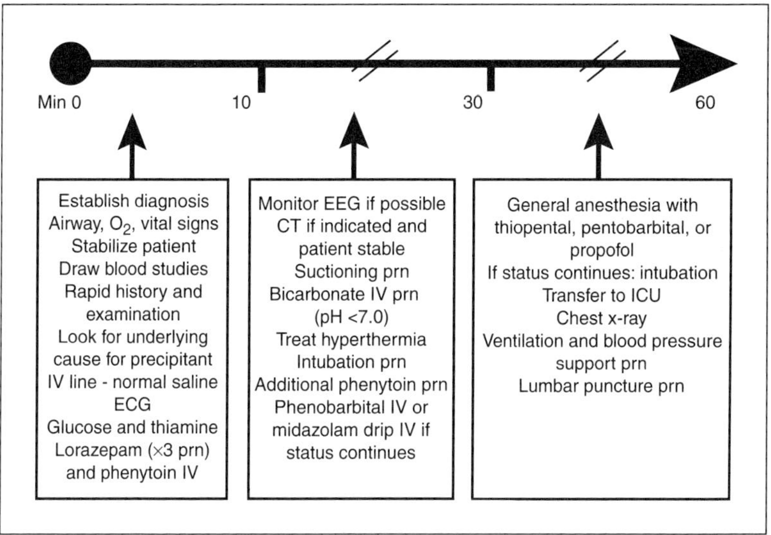

FIGURE 8.1 Timeline for management of convulsive status epilepticus. (ECG = electrocardiogram; EEG = electroencephalography; ICU = intensive care unit.)

Goals of Management of Status

- Immediate and continued stabilization of vital signs and support of cardiopulmonary function
- Preservation of neurons (stop seizures)
- Treatment of causes and precipitants (e.g., meningitis, stroke, hyponatremia)
- Prevention of medical complications of status (e.g., myoglobinuria and renal failure, aspiration, disseminated intravascular coagulation)
- Prevention of immediate and future recurrence of seizures and status

Special Considerations

- Severe hyponatremia may require treatment with hypertonic saline, but rapidity of correction of hyponatremia must proceed according to guidelines to prevent central pontine myelinolysis.
- Treatment of status due to isonicotinic acid hydrazide (isoniazid) intoxication should include large doses of pyridoxine IV.
- Physostigmine can be given for tricyclic antidepressant and other atropinic agent intoxication.
- Domoic acid intoxication, occurring in outbreaks due to eating contaminated mussels, has rarely caused intractable status.

- Eclampsia should be treated as outlined in the section on pregnancy (see Chapter 7).
- Porphyria is a rare cause of SE; its management is discussed in etiologies of epilepsy (see Chapter 3).

Common Errors in Management of Status Epilepticus

- Misdiagnosis (e.g., pseudoseizures, decerebrate spasms)
- Missing and not treating underlying cause (e.g., meningitis, hypoglycemia)
- Not correcting hyperthermia, hypoxia, hyperkalemia, severe acidosis
- Intubating too late
- Wrong route of drug administration (e.g., phenytoin IM)
- Inadequate drug dosage (common error in someone already receiving AEDs)
- Excessive delay in switching to another drug or in instituting general anesthesia
- Delay in initiation of maintenance AED therapy after treatment of SE
- Overtreatment of myoclonic or EEG status after global cerebral hypoxia or ischemia due to cardiac arrest

Partial Motor Status Epilepticus

- Has a number of etiologies, including stroke, head trauma, cerebral infection, cerebral hypoxia, and occasionally metabolic abnormalities (sometimes combined with underlying subtle structural abnormalities).
- EEG in many cases shows PLEDs.
- *Epilepsy partialis continua* is a specific category that is not due to acute brain disease and does not require aggressive initial treatment.
- The aggressiveness of management depends on the potential adverse effects of the seizures. For example, older patients may have cardiac or respiratory compromise from ongoing vigorous focal motor seizures, and patients with acute strokes and focal motor status risk worsening ischemic damage.
- Treatment is similar to generalized convulsive SE with less urgency for generalized anesthesia.
- An oral loading dose of clobazam (1 mg/kg) may be used in patients not responding to IV benzodiazepines and phenytoin (Corman et al., 1998).
- In most patients, SE ceases spontaneously after 48–72 hours, once the acute brain insult has settled or specific treatment for metabolic or infectious etiologies has been given.

Prognosis of Status

- In 1970, Aicardi and Chevrie found an 11% mortality in infants and children, one-half due to the SE itself.
- In Goulon et al.'s 1985 series from France, of 282 adult cases of status, only two deaths were attributed to the SE itself. Mortality rates in SE were 7% in patients with preexisting epilepsy and 47% in patients with de novo SE.

- In 1989, Phillips and Shanahan found a 6% mortality in 218 episodes of childhood status.
- In 1994, Shorvon reviewed 15 series of SE, representing 1,689 cases, and calculated an 18% mortality. In 89% of cases, death was related to the underlying CNS or systemic disease causing the status rather than the SE itself.
- In a prospective population-based study of SE conducted in 1996 by DeLorenzo et al., there was a 22% overall mortality in 166 patients (204 episodes): 3% mortality in children, 13% in young adults, 26% in adults, and 38% in older patients.
- Lowenstein and Alldredge reported in 1998 that if SE persists for 4 hours despite treatment, mortality is less than or equal to 50%; if status is not controlled in 12 hours or less, mortality rises to more than 80%.

Suggested Reading

Aicardi JF, Chevrie JJ. Convulsive status epilepticus in infants and children: a study of 239 cases. Epilepsia 1970;11:187-197.

Aminoff MJ, Simon RP. Status epilepticus: causes, clinical features and consequences in 98 patients. Am J Med 1980;69:657-665.

Berkovic SF, Guberman A, Hipola D, et al. Valproate prevents the recurrence of absence status. Neurology 1989;39:1294-1297.

Bone RC. Treatment of convulsive status epilepticus. JAMA 1993;270:854-859.

Chang CWJ, Bleck TP. Status epilepticus. Neurol Clin 1995;13:529-548.

Cockerell OC, Rothwell J, Thompson PD, et al. Clinical and physiological features of epilepsy partialis continua. Cases ascertained in the U.K. Brain 1996;119:393-407.

Corman C, Guberman A, Benavente O. Clobazam in partial status epilepticus. Seizure 1998;7:243-247.

Delgado-Escueta AV, Wasterlain CG, Treiman DM, et al. (eds). Status Epilepticus: Mechanisms of Brain Damage and Treatment. Advances in Neurology (Vol. 34). New York: Raven, 1983.

DeLorenzo RJ, Hauser WA, Towne AR, et al. A prospective, population-based epidemiologic study of status epilepticus in Richmond, Virginia. Neurology 1996;46:1029-1035.

DeLorenzo RJ, Pellock JM, Towne AR, et al. Epidemiology of status epilepticus. J Clin Neurophysiol 1995;12:316-325.

DeLorenzo RJ, Towne AR, Pellock JM, Ko D. Status epilepticus in children, adults, and the elderly. Epilepsia 1992;33(Suppl 4):S15-S25.

Dreifuss FE, Rosman NP, Cloyd JC, et al. A comparison of rectal diazepam gel and placebo for acute reactive seizures. N Engl J Med 1998;338:1869-1875.

Giroud M, Gras D, Escousse A, et al. Use of injectable valproic acid in status epilepticus: a pilot study. Drug Invest 1995;5:154-159.

Goulon M, Lévy-Alcover MA, Nouailhat F. État de mal épileptique de l'adulte: étude épidémiologique et clinique en réanimation. Rev Electroencéphal Neurophysiol Clin 1985;15: 277-285.

Grimes D, Guberman A. De novo aphasic status epilepticus. Epilepsia 1997;38:945-949.

Guberman A, Cantu-Reyna G, Broughton R. Non-convulsive generalized status epilepticus: clinical features, neuropsychological testing and long-term follow-up. Neurology 1986;36:1284-1291.

Jagoda A, Riggio S (eds). Management of seizures in the emergency department. Emerg Med Clin North Am 1994;12:895-1139.

Kaplan PW. Nonconvulsive status epilepticus. Semin Neurol 1996;16:33-40.

Krishnamurthy KB, Drislane FW. Relapse and survival after barbiturate anesthetic treatment of refractory status epilepticus. Epilepsia 1996;37:863-867.

Krumholz A, Sung GY, Fisher RS, et al. Complex partial status epilepticus accompanied by serious morbidity and mortality. Neurology 1995;45:1499-1504.

Kumar A, Bleck TP. Intravenous midazolam for the treatment of refractory status epilepticus. Crit Care Med 1992;20:483-488.

Leppik IE (ed). Status epilepticus in perspective. Neurology 1990;40(Suppl 2):1-51.

Leppik IE, Derivan AT, Homan RW, et al. Double-blind study of lorazepam and diazepam in status epilepticus. JAMA 1983;249:1432-1454.

Lowenstein DH, Alldredge BK. Status epilepticus. N Engl J Med 1998;338:970-976.

Martin PJ, Millac PAH. Status epilepticus: management and outcome of 107 episodes. Seizure 1994;3:107-113.

Novak G, Maytal J, Alshansky A, et al. Risk factors for status epilepticus in children with symptomatic epilepsy. Neurology 1997;49:533-537.

Parent JM, Lowenstein DH. Treatment of refractory generalized status epilepticus with continuous infusion of midazolam. Neurology 1994;44:1837-1840.

Pellock JM. Status epilepticus in children: update and review. J Child Neurol 1994;9(Suppl 2):S27-S35.

Phillips SA, Shanahan RJ. Etiology and mortality of status epilepticus in children. Arch Neurol 1989;46:74-76.

Ramsay RE, Wilder BJ, Uthman BM, et al. Intramuscular fosphenytoin (Cerebyx) in patients requiring a loading dose of phenytoin. Epilepsy Res 1997;28:181-187.

Rao VK, Feldman PD, Dibbell DG. Extravasation injury to the hand by intravenous phenytoin. J Neurosurg 1988;68:967-969.

Rashkin MC, Younge C, Panovich P. Pentobarbital treatment of refractory status epilepticus. Neurology 1987;37:500-502.

Scholtes FB, Renier WO, Meinardi H. Generalized convulsive status epilepticus: causes, therapy and outcome in 346 patients. Epilepsia 1994;35:1104-1112.

Scholtes FB, Renier WO, Meinardi H. Simple partial status epilepticus: causes, treatment, and outcome in 47 patients. J Neurol Neurosurg Psychiatry 1996;61:90-92.

Shaner DM, McCurdy SA, Herring MO, et al. Treatment of status epilepticus: a prospective comparison of diazepam and phenytoin compared with phenobarbital and optional phenytoin. Neurology 1988;38:202-207.

Shinnar S, Pellock JM, Moshé SL, et al. In whom does status epilepticus occur: age-related differences in children. Epilepsia 1997;38:907-914.

Shorvon S. Status Epilepticus: Its Clinical Features and Treatment in Children and Adults. Cambridge, UK: Cambridge University Press, 1994.

Shorvon S. The outcome of tonic-clonic status epilepticus. Curr Opin Neurol 1994;7:93-95.

Simkins RT, Barkley GL. Status epilepticus in adolescents and adults. Curr Neurol 1995;15:61-99.

Stecker MM, Kramer TH, Raps EC, et al. Treatment of refractory status epilepticus with propofol: clinical and pharmacokinetic findings. Epilepsia 1998;39:18-26.

Treiman DM, Walton NY, Kendrick C. A progressive sequence of electrographic changes during generalized convulsive status epilepticus. Epilepsy Res 1990;5:49-60.

Walker MC. The epidemiology and management of status epilepticus. Curr Opin Neurol 1998;11:149-154.

Wilder BJ (ed). The use of parenteral antiepileptic drugs and the role for fosphenytoin. Neurology 1996;46:(Suppl 1):S1-S28.

9 Surgical Treatment

- Surgical treatment for epilepsy is generally considered for patients with refractory partial seizures.
- Ten percent to 15% of patients with refractory seizures may be surgical candidates.
- The tendency to operate on intractable patients with partial epilepsy has grown, and surgery on children has increased in the hope of averting the long-term consequences of uncontrolled epilepsy during the formative years.
- The definition of *intractable* is not generally agreed on, and in some cases, despite good seizure control, surgery is considered because even occasional seizures are particularly psychosocially disabling for the patient or intolerable side effects of AEDs are present.
- All available clinical and testing data are routinely used and combined to localize the site of seizure origin.
- The aim of surgery is to remove the focus of origin of the seizures or to prevent spread of the seizure discharge. After successful surgery, some patients who formerly experienced secondarily generalized tonic-clonic seizures or complex partial seizures experience only auras.
- Some cases with bilateral or multiple foci may be candidates for surgery if the vast majority of seizures can be localized to a single focus.

Presurgical Evaluation

Patient Selection

Surgical candidates must have the following:

- Medically intractable epileptic seizures
- Seizures that are significantly socially disabling
- Absence of severe fixed neurologic and cognitive deficits in addition to seizures
- Well-established seizure pattern spanning at least 1–2 years
- Identifiable focus of origin for the majority of the seizures (except for callosotomy candidates)
- A relatively low risk of severe neurologic deficit (e.g., aphasia) if surgery of the focus is being considered

- Motivation and willingness to cooperate with the investigations, surgery, and follow-up; well-motivated family
- Absence of medical contraindications to surgery
- Adequate social support system

Clinical Evaluation

- Establish that the patient has epilepsy and identify seizure type by carefully evaluating patient history.
- Establish that patient has true medical intractability after the patient has had adequate therapy trials (efficacy failure of two or three first-line drugs in adequate doses generally indicates medical intractability).
- Determine impact of epilepsy on patient's quality of life.
- Assess for presence of drug toxicity.
- Assess patient for focal neurologic signs that may indicate site of focal pathology.
- Obtain detailed seizure description from patient and observers.
- Assess social and psychiatric aspects of patient's epilepsy. Severe psychosis may be a relative contraindication.
- Assess patient's degree of motivation and understanding of and willingness to accept the risk-benefit ratio.
- Screen for contraindications to surgery, which include degenerative diseases, serious intercurrent medical illnesses, or epilepsy syndromes that have a high probability of remission.

Electroencephalography

- Interictal recordings (may or may not correspond to ictal focus).
- Ictal recordings to document seizure onset.
- EEG/video telemetry monitoring is required in the majority of patients, often on an inpatient basis over several days.
- Intracranial EEG recordings with epidural electrodes, subdural strip electrodes, or (rarely) intracerebral (depth) electrodes if difficulty in localizing seizure onset or discordant data exist (e.g., scalp EEG points to one site and neuroimaging to another).
- AEDs often discontinued during period of EEG recordings to hasten occurrence of seizures.
- Intraoperative electrocorticography.

Neuroimaging

- MRI is indicated in all surgical candidates.
- Assessment for hippocampal volume and T2 relaxation times, other focal pathologies, and dual pathologies.
- PET and postictal SPECT, when available, may provide useful data in selected cases.
- Functional MRI, when available, may be useful for localization.

Neuropsychological Psychiatric Assessment

Objectives of neuropsychological assessment include the following:

- To document areas of functional deficit
- For speech lateralization studies (e.g., Wada test, dichotic listening) to determine cerebral dominance
- To predict neuropsychological deficits (e.g., memory) that might occur as a result of surgery

Psychiatric assessment may be indicated in patients who have psychological/psychiatric symptoms in association with their epilepsy.

Surgical Procedures

- *Anterior temporal lobectomy* is the most frequently performed surgical procedure. Anterior temporal lobe resection extends 4.0–5.5 cm behind the temporal pole. Resection includes the amygdala, anterior hippocampus, and anterior temporal neocortex. In many cases, patients are awake during the surgery to map functional areas such as language centers.
- Selective *amygdalohippocampectomy* is performed in patients with focal pathology such as mesial-temporal sclerosis or developmental tumors confined to mesial-temporal structures. There is less risk of visual field defects, dysphasia, and possibly memory impairment. If seizure control is not satisfactory, more extensive resection can be considered.
- *Lesionectomy*: removal of epileptogenic lesions—temporal or extratemporal.
  - Most frequent pathologies include low-grade gliomas such as gangliomas or dysembryoplastic neuroepithelial tumors, vascular anomalies (e.g., cavernous angiomas), post-traumatic scars, focal encephalitis, cortical dysplasias, and neuronal migration disorders.
  - In presence of dual pathology (e.g., mesial-temporal sclerosis and dysplastic lesions), the lesion responsible or most responsible for the epilepsy must be identified.
- In patients with generalized seizures, an anterior two-thirds *corpus callosotomy* can be performed initially; if necessary, it can be extended to a complete callosotomy in a subsequent procedure. Corpus callosotomy (anterior or complete) is generally a palliative procedure directed to prevent seizure spread from one hemisphere to the other; it is most frequently indicated for patients who have drop (atonic) seizures in the absence of any resectable lesion. Patients often have cryptogenic or symptomatic generalized seizure disorders such as Lennox-Gastaut syndrome.
- *Hemispherectomy* should be considered in patients with medical intractability due to severe unilateral pathologies, as may occur with congenital malformations, Rasmussen's encephalitis, Sturge-Weber syndrome, pre- or perinatal injuries, cerebral palsy secondary to vascular etiologies, or widespread unilateral EEG abnormalities. Various surgical techniques are used, including functional hemispherectomy and hemidecortication. Hemispherectomy should

only be considered in patients who have a severe, contralateral neurologic deficit with no useful hand or fine finger movements.
- *Multiple subpial transections* to prevent the propagation of seizure activity can be performed if the epileptic focus is in an eloquent area of brain (e.g., precentral motor strip) that cannot be removed without a major functional deficit. Results are generally less satisfactory than with resective surgery. Possible indications include partial motor or sensory seizures, Landau-Kleffner syndrome, local cortical dysplasia, epilepsia partialis continua, and Rasmussen's encephalitis.

Goals of Therapy

- To improve the patient's quality of life by maximizing seizure control and minimizing drug adverse effects
- To reduce psychosocial disability
- To reduce medical morbidity
- To minimize surgical neurologic deficit

Results of Surgical Treatment

- Classification of seizure outcome after epilepsy surgery as proposed by Engel (1993) (modified):

I. Class I
  A. Completely seizure-free
  B. Auras only
II. Class II
  A. Rare seizures
  B. Nocturnal seizures only
III. Class III: worthwhile decrease in seizures
IV. Class IV
  A. No significant seizure reduction
  B. Seizures worse

- Results of surgical treatment for focal lesions depend on the nature of the underlying pathology and its location.
- Best prognosis for mesial-temporal sclerosis with hippocampal atrophy, temporal lobe low-grade gliomas, or developmental tumors: 70–80% of patients become seizure-free. Another 20–25% of patients have a significant but incomplete reduction in seizures. The outcome with extratemporal resection is less satisfactory, with only 30–50% of patients becoming seizure-free. The least favorable prognosis is with extensive cortical dysplastic lesions, because it is difficult to resect all of the epileptogenic zone.

- Improvement may continue for years after surgery.
- With functional hemispherectomy, 75–80% of patients become seizure-free and have improved behavior. Patients retain the ability to walk.
- Corpus callosotomy may significantly reduce drop attacks in 50–75% of patients.
- Psychosocial improvement after successful surgery generally occurs, but some patients have difficulty adjusting to life without seizures. Their longstanding lack of life or vocational skills may prevent significant improvement in their postsurgery quality of life.
- Overall risk of severe neurologic complications from epilepsy surgery is approximately 1%. The types and incidences of complications depend on the type and extent of the surgical procedure. Many of the complications are perioperative, including brain abscesses and, rarely, focal neurologic strokelike deficits. With left temporal lobectomy, a mild verbal memory deficit may occur. Depression can occur after surgery and last for several months. Late development of psychosis has been seen (rarely) years after successful temporal lobectomy.
- Whether and when to discontinue AEDs after successful surgery is controversial and is generally decided on an individual patient basis.

Cost-Effectiveness

- Benefit ratio may be highest for children.
- By several years postsurgery, surgical therapy may be more cost-effective than medical therapy.

Reoperation

- Considered in patients in whom adequate results were not achieved by first procedure, which may have been a small resection.
- Some patients who have had selective amygdalohippocampectomy may benefit from a more traditional anterior temporal resection.
- Patients who have had an initial anterior corpus callosotomy may benefit from a complete callosotomy.
- Of reoperated patients, 30–40% become seizure-free, and 30% have a significant improvement.
- Temporal lobe reoperations generally are more successful than extratemporal reoperations.
- Complications from reoperation are higher than with the first procedure.

Vagus Nerve Stimulation

Vagus nerve stimulation is a relatively new surgical approach to intractable epilepsy in patients who have not responded to drug treatment or traditional epilepsy surgery or who are not candidates for (or who do not wish to undergo) intracranial surgery. Its place in epilepsy management is still being established.

Technique

- Pacemaker-like device delivers electrical stimulation to the left vagus nerve.
- Mechanism of antiepileptic effect is unknown but presumably acts by changing brain electrical activity, neurotransmitter function, or both.
- NeuroCybernetics Prosthesis (Cyberonics, Inc., Webster, TX): System includes battery-powered generator (programmable chip, Li pacemaker battery), electrodes, programming wand (attaches to laptop computer by serial port), software, magnets, and tunneling tool.
- Two helical stimulating electrodes and an anchor electrode attach to the left vagus nerve in the neck. They are connected to the generator implanted subcutaneously in the upper chest below the clavicle.
- Stimulation protocol can be changed. Most common is 1.25- to 1.50-mA current, 30-Hz, 500-ms pulse width, 30 seconds of stimulation alternating with 5 minutes of no stimulation.
- The system is programmed by a magnetic wand held over the generator. The wand is connected to the computer, and software allows programming.
- A magnet carried by the patient can be held briefly over the generator to administer an extra charge (e.g., when aura is felt), or, if taped over the generator, will deactivate the system temporarily. Activation of the magnet at the beginning of the seizure or during the aura may abort, shorten, or reduce the intensity of the seizure.
- The generator unit must be replaced when the battery wears out (after approximately 3–5 years).

Efficacy

- Approximately one-third to one-half of patients have greater than 50% seizure reduction when used in addition to previous AEDs. Rarely, patients have complete seizure control.
- Appears to work for a broad variety of seizure types.
- Effective in adults and children.
- Efficacy may improve over time in a given patient.

Adverse Effects

- Hoarseness (postoperative, transient, intermittent during stimulation)
- Throat pain or paresthesias
- Coughing
- Hiccoughs
- Dyspnea

- Perioperative infection
- Recurrent laryngeal nerve paralysis, platysma paralysis (both rare)

Advantages and Disadvantages

Advantages

- Minimal side effects, no cognitive or behavioral side effects
- Possibility of abortive as well as preventive treatment
- Avoids compliance problems
- Appears to work for a wide variety of seizure types
- Reduces seizure severity and frequency

Disadvantages

- Criteria for selection of patients most likely to benefit are not well established
- Costly
- Invasive (surgical procedure)
- Needs replacement after battery wears out in 3-5 years
- Unproven efficacy when used as monotherapy (i.e., without AEDs)

Suggested Reading

Surgical Treatment of Epilepsy

Abou-Khalil BAE, Andermann F. Temporal lobe epilepsy after prolonged febrile convulsions: excellent outcome after surgical treatment. Epilepsia 1993;34:878-883.

Arruda F, Cendes F, Andermann F, et al. Mesial atrophy and outcome after amygdalohippocampectomy or temporal lobe removal. Ann Neurol 1996;40:446-450.

Boling W, Olivier A. The current state of epilepsy surgery. Curr Opin Neurol 1998;11: 155-161.

Chugani HT, Shields WD, Shewmon DA, et al. Infantile spasms: I. PET identifies focal cortical dysgenesis in cryptogenic cases for surgical treatment. Ann Neurol 1990;27:406-413.

Devinsky O, Pacia S. Epilepsy surgery. Neurol Clin 1993;11:951-971.

Engel J Jr (ed). Surgical Treatment of the Epilepsies. New York: Raven, 1993.

Engel J Jr. Epilepsy surgery. Curr Opin Neurol 1994;7:140-147.

Engel JE. Update on surgical treatment of the epilepsies. Neurology 1993;43:1612-1617.

Fish DR, Smith SJ, Quesney LF, et al. Surgical treatment of children with medically intractable frontal or temporal lobe epilepsy: results and highlights of 40 years' experience. Epilepsia 1993;34:244-247.

George RE, Mizhari EM, Fishman MA. Surgical treatment of epilepsy in children. Curr Neurol 1993;13:229-264.

Holmes GL. Surgery for intractable seizures in infancy and childhood. Neurology 1993; 3(Suppl 5):S28-S37.

NIH Consensus Panel. Consensus conference on surgery for epilepsy. JAMA 1990;264: 729-733.

Palmini A, Andermann F, Dubeau F, et al. Occipitotemporal epilepsies: evaluation of selected patients requiring depth electrodes studies and rationale for surgical approaches. Epilepsia 1993;34:84-96.

Palmini A, Gambardella A, Andermann F, et al. Operative strategies for patients with cortical dysplastic lesions and intractable epilepsy. Epilepsia 1994;35(Suppl 6):S57-S71.

Polkey CE, Binnie CD. Assessment and selection of candidates for surgical treatment of epilepsy. Epilepsia 1995;36(Suppl 1):S41-S45.

Riggio S. Frontal lobe epilepsy: clinical syndromes and presurgical evaluation. J Epilepsy 1995;8:178-189.

Sawhney S, Robertson IJ, Polkey CE, et al. Multiple subpial transection: a review of 21 cases. J Neurol Neurosurg Psychiatry 1995;58:344-349.

Smith MC. Multiple subpial transection in patients with extratemporal epilepsy. Epilepsia 1998;39(Suppl 4):S81-S89.

Smith SJ, Andermann F, Villemure JG, et al. Functional hemispherectomy: EEG findings, spiking from isolated brain postoperatively, and prediction of outcome. Neurology 1991;41:1790-1794.

Spencer SS. Surgical options for uncontrolled epilepsy. Neurol Clin 1986;4:669-695.

Spencer SS. The relative contributions of MRI, SPECT and PET in epilepsy surgery. Epilepsia 1994;35(Suppl 6):S72-S89.

Spencer SS. MRI and epilepsy surgery. Neurology 1995;45:1248-1250.

Spencer SS. Long-term outcome after epilepsy surgery. Epilepsia 1996;37:807-813.

Sperling M, O'Connor MI, Saykin AJ, et al. Temporal lobectomy for refractory epilepsy. JAMA 1996;276:470-475.

Vickrey BG, Hays RD, Rausch R, et al. Outcomes in 248 patients who had diagnostic evaluations for epilepsy surgery. Lancet 1995;346:1145-1149.

Wass CT, Rajala MM, Hughes JM, et al. Long term follow-up of patients treated surgically for medically intractable epilepsy. Mayo Clin Proc 1996;71:1105-1113.

Zentner J, Hufnagel A, Wolf HK, et al. Surgical treatment of temporal lobe epilepsy: clinical, radiological and histopathological findings in 178 patients. J Neurol Neurosurg Psychiatry 1995;58:666-673.

Vagus Nerve Stimulation

Handforth A, DeGiorgio CM, Schacter SC, et al. Vagus nerve stimulation therapy for partial-onset seizures. a randomized active-control trial. Neurology 1998;51:48-55.

McLachlan R. Vagus nerve stimulation for intractable epilepsy: a review. J Clin Neurophysiol 1997;14:358-368.

Schacter SC, Saper CB. Vagus nerve stimulation. Epilepsia 1998;39:677-686.

Takaya M, Terry WJ, Naritoku DK. Vagus nerve stimulation induces a sustained anticonvulsant effect. Epilepsia 1996;37:1111-1116.

10 Psychosocial Aspects

The psychosocial consequences of epilepsy are a major component of the disability associated with the condition; they often outweigh the physical consequences of the seizures and their treatment (Figure 10.1). The origin of the psychological and psychiatric consequences is multifactorial and may include

- Effects of ictal and subclinical epileptic discharges on limbic neurons and circuits
- Effects of underlying pathology causing epilepsy and also behavioral changes, possibly through neurotransmitter disturbances
- Social consequences of epilepsy producing disturbed interpersonal relations and interfering with normal psychosocial development
- Effects of AEDs

The *stigmatization* of epilepsy has historical roots (e.g., equating epilepsy with "possession by the devil," associating epilepsy with violent criminal behavior) and often leads to low self-esteem and social isolation. *Fear* of seizures by the patient may be related to fear of loss of control, fear of injury or death related to a seizure, or fear of peri-ictal or postictal dysphoric states. *Loss of independence* is a common consequence that may be related to factors including overprotection, inability to drive, and having to take medication.

Depression is the most common psychiatric problem seen in epileptic patients. It may be periodic and related to seizures. Suicide risk is increased at least fivefold in epileptic patients compared to the normal population (for which suicide risk is less than 1%). Antidepressants that are least likely to lower seizure threshold are doxepin, alprazolam, desipramine, fluoxetine, sertraline, fluvoxamine, and venlafaxine. The selective serotonin reuptake inhibitors are the antidepressants of choice. Valproate and carbamazepine may be useful for their mood stabilizing effects.

Interictal personality traits have been studied extensively in epileptic patients. A clustering of certain traits typically seen in epileptic patients was proposed by Bear and Fedio (1977), but this profile is by no means common in or specific to the epileptic patient. The described traits are a preoccupation with religious and philosophical matters; viscosity; circumstantial concern with

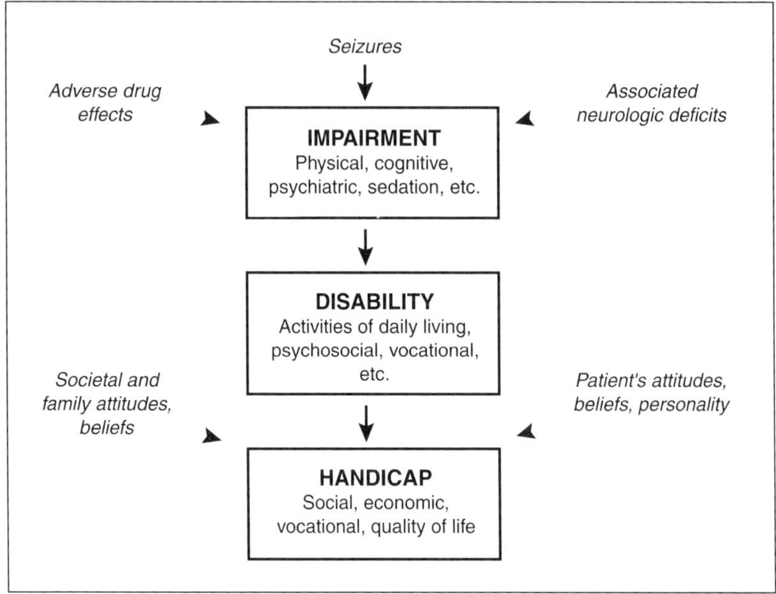

FIGURE 10.1 Some determinants of quality of life in epilepsy patients.

details; humorless, sober affect; irritability ("short fuse"); excessive emotionality; hypergraphia and hyposexuality.

Violence and Epilepsy

- The relationship between violence and epilepsy has been much debated and has legal implications.
- *Violence* can be defined as physical aggression, either provoked or unprovoked, directed toward a person with the intent or seeming intent to injure or kill.
- An unproven correlation between epilepsy in general and interictal violent behavior exists, despite the fact that prison surveys show a two- to fourfold increase in epileptic persons as compared to the general population.
- The most common form of violence seen during a seizure is combativeness during postictal confusion, which is an automatism in reaction to attempts to restrain or impede the patient.
- Directed violence as part of an epileptic seizure occurs extremely rarely; when it does, it is brief, impulsive, and uncoordinated and does not consist of a series of planned, deliberate actions.
- Suggested criteria (Delgado-Escueta et al., 1981) for attributing a criminal violent act to an epileptic seizure:

- A definite diagnosis of epilepsy to be established by at least one neurologist with expertise in epilepsy.
- The presence of an epileptic automatism to be established by history and EEG or video monitoring.
- The presence of aggression during an automatism, documented by a video recording and correlated with EEG ictal activity.
- The recorded ictal aggressive act should be typical of the patient's spontaneous seizures.
- The neurologist, using clinical judgment, should attest to the possibility that the crime was part of a seizure.

Psychosis in Epilepsy

Psychosis in epilepsy is seen in five main contexts:

- Postictal psychosis or delirium.
  - Often follows a closely spaced series of complex partial or generalized tonic-clonic seizures (e.g., in patients in whom AEDs have been withdrawn for presurgical workup)
  - Usually manifests as an agitated delirium with paranoid ideation and, at times, hallucinations
  - Usually lasts for 2-3 days
- Interictal schizophreniform psychosis.
  - Seen in 5-10% of patients, usually with temporolimbic epilepsy
  - Usually in longstanding epilepsy
  - Differs from classic schizophrenia in that premorbid personality is usually normal, family history is usually negative, affect is relatively well preserved, and there is less long-term deterioration
  - May have a higher incidence with foreign tissue lesions
- *Alternating psychosis* (forced normalization of the EEG) is rare and implies a reciprocal relationship between the degree of seizure control and psychiatric status. When seizures are controlled and the EEG is normalized, psychotic behavior emerges. Ethosuximide was associated with this state in early descriptions, but other AEDs can have the same effect when seizures are controlled.
- Psychosis can emerge as a late complication, years after successful temporal lobectomy.
- *AED-induced psychosis* or severe depression has been described in 2-4% of patients treated with vigabatrin and, rarely, with other AEDs such as topiramate or clobazam. The incidence with vigabatrin may be reduced by slow titration (not more than 500 mg per week); by using the drug cautiously in patients with a significant psychiatric history; and by warning patients and families to watch for prodromal behavioral changes such as withdrawal, irritability, or suspiciousness, which should lead to discontinuation of the drug.

Major tranquilizers that are least likely to lower seizure threshold include thioridazine, pimozide, risperidone, and haloperidol.

TABLE 10.1 Potential Effects of Antiepileptic Drugs on Cognitive Function and Behavior

Antiepileptic Drug	*Cognition*	*Behavior*
Carbamazepine	Minimal	Mood stabilizer
Phenytoin	Impairs	Not clear
Phenobarbital	Impairs	Depression
Valproic acid	Minimal	Mood stabilizer
Clobazam	Minimal	Depression/irritability
Clonazepam	Impairs	? Mood stabilizer
Vigabatrin	Minimal	Psychosis/depression
Gabapentin	Minimal	Minimal
Lamotrigine	Minimal	Minimal
Topiramate	Impairs	Minimal, psychosis reported
Tiagabine	Minimal	Minimal
Felbamate	Minimal	Minimal

Other Effects of Antiepileptic Drugs

- AED-induced behavior changes of a less severe degree, including irritability, withdrawal, and hypomania, are commonly seen with a wide variety of AEDs, especially in children with cognitive impairment.
- Table 10.1 contains a summary of potential AED effects on cognition and behavior.

Quality of Life

- Health-related *quality of life* (QOL) is a concept increasingly applied to individual patient and therapeutic trial outcomes in epilepsy.
- The following domains of QOL have been proposed by the World Health Organization:
  - Physical health
  - Psychological health
  - Level of independence
  - Social relationships
  - Environment (includes physical environment, work satisfaction, health and social care, transportation)
- QOL measures use patient (rather than physician) perception to determine therapeutic outcome or simple measures such as seizure count or seizure severity.
- A commonly used instrument is the Quality of Life in Epilepsy-31 Questionnaire or its scaled-down, 10-item version, the QOLIE-10 Questionnaire, which looks at the following issues (see Figure 10.1):

- Energy
- Feelings of depression
- Driving ability
- Memory difficulties
- Work limitations
- Social limitations
- Physical effects of AEDs
- Mental effects of AEDs
- Fear of seizures
- Overall QOL

Practical Advice for the Epileptic Patient

The following advice is for patients who are having ongoing seizures, especially with impairment of consciousness.

- Avoid sleep deprivation and excessive alcohol use.
- Avoid jobs that entail working on heights or near heavy machinery, flames, burners, or molten material. Certain careers such as fire fighting, airplane piloting, bus driving, and truck driving are not recommended.
- Never swim alone. Take showers sitting on a low stool rather than baths.
- Microwave cooking is preferable to stovetop cooking.
- Most sports are permitted, but those in which a sudden loss of consciousness would be dangerous, such as sky diving, hang gliding, para sailing, bungie jumping, competitive cycling, rapid downhill skiing, mountain and rock climbing, surfing, and scuba diving, are best avoided. Sports in which head injuries are common, such as boxing, are not recommended.
- When a dose of medication is missed, it should be added to the next dose.
- With phenytoin treatment, meticulous dental and gum care, as recommended by a dental hygienist or dentist, is necessary to prevent excessive tooth decay and gum problems.
- Laws concerning driving vary, but they generally do not allow driving a motor vehicle for 1–2 years after the last seizure. Exceptions may exist for seizures that are strictly nocturnal or simple partial or for those that are related to discontinuation of anticonvulsant medication on a physician's advice.
- A medical alert bracelet or necklace should be worn.
- First aid for a seizure consists of the following:
  - Protecting the patient's head and body from injury.
  - Removing dentures, excessive secretions, and other foreign material from the mouth after the tonic and clonic phases.
  - Turning the patient to the semiprone position in the postictal period to prevent aspiration and blockage of the nasopharynx.
  - It is unnecessary to take the patient to the hospital in the postictal period after one or two uncomplicated seizures. However, if three or more seizures occur in a brief time or the patient does not regain full consciousness within a few hours, he or she should be seen by a physician.

Driving Issues

- Accident rates among epileptic patients are difficult to calculate, but relative risks are generally 1.5–2.0 times higher than those among the general public.
- Accident risk may depend on factors other than seizures, such as associated neurologic handicaps, effects of medication, and lack of driving experience.
- Withdrawal of driving privileges is frequently a major handicap that impacts independence and self-esteem in adolescents, limits employment options, and interferes with daily functioning, especially in older patients and patients who live in rural settings.
- Driving regulations vary from country to country and from state to state (within the United States) or province to province (in Canada).
- In most states and provinces, a seizure-free interval of 1 year is required to drive, although 10 states have no specified seizure-free interval. Mandatory continued reporting is required at varying intervals. A commercial license (e.g., to drive passengers or transport materials) is generally not allowed as long as the patient is on AEDs.
- Mandatory reporting by physicians is required in California, Delaware, Nevada, New Jersey, Oregon, and Pennsylvania in the United States and in Manitoba, Ontario, Prince Edward Island, Newfoundland, New Brunswick, Northwest Territories, and Yukon in Canada. Most physicians believe the requirement for mandatory reporting puts an unfair burden on the physician and interferes with the physician-patient relationship, encouraging patients to lie or conceal important information about their seizures or, in the worst case, avoiding physician care altogether for fear of having their licenses revoked.
- State-by-state regulations pertaining to driving and epilepsy are available through state licensing authorities or the Epilepsy Foundation of America (http://www.efa.org).
- Various medical groups have appealed to governments and licensing agencies to
  - Put the legal and moral responsibility for reporting the epilepsy on the patient.
  - Determine ability to drive on a case-by-case basis rather than making a blanket rule for all patients diagnosed with epilepsy.
  - Protect physicians who report patients whom they consider unsafe to drive from legal action.
  - Apply the driving laws for epilepsy patients and other patient groups with medical conditions that could affect driving in a consistent fashion.
  - Establish a system for patients who feel their driving privileges have been unfairly withdrawn to make appeals.
  - Distinguish between regular licenses and special licenses for driving transport vehicles and public transportation vehicles or operating heavy equipment.
- Guidelines and laws concerning driving and epilepsy should cover the following points and situations:
  - Seizure-free interval required for driving (generally 1 year)

- First seizure in a previously neurologically normal individual (3-6 months without driving may be reasonable)
- First seizure in a previously neurologically abnormal individual or one with a newly acquired neurologic insult such as stroke or brain surgery (6 months without driving may be reasonable)
- Strictly nocturnal seizures over a relatively long period of observation (e.g., 5 years)
- Simple partial seizures without loss of consciousness or generalization and without significant motor impairment over a prolonged period (e.g., 5 years)
- Period without driving required following withdrawal of AEDs after a seizure-free interval of 2 years or more (3-6 months may be reasonable)
- Patient compliance and reliablity (e.g., taking AEDs properly, avoidance of excessive alcohol use, honest reporting of seizures, avoidance of driving when overtired) to be taken into account

Suggested Reading

Bear DM, Fedio P. Quantitative analysis of interictal behavior in temporal lobe epilepsy. Arch Neurol 1977;34:454-467.

Collaborative Group for Epidemiology of Epilepsy. Adverse reactions to antiepileptic drugs. A follow-up study of 355 patients with chronic antiepileptic drug treatment. Epilepsia 1988;29:787-793.

Commission of Pediatrics of the ILAE. Restrictions for children with epilepsy. Epilepsia 1997;38:1054-1056.

Cramer JA. A clinometric approach to assessing quality of life in epilepsy. Epilepsia 1993;34:S8-S13.

Delgado-Escueta AV, Mattson RH, King L, et al. Special report. The nature of aggression during epileptic seizures. N Engl J Med 1981;305:711-716.

Devinsky O. Clinical uses of the Quality-of-Life in Epilepsy Inventory. Epilepsia 1993;34 (Suppl 4):S39-S44.

Devinsky O, Penry JK. Quality of life in epilepsy: the clinician's view. Epilepsia 1993;34 (Suppl 4):S4-S7.

Devinsky O, Theodore WH (eds). Epilepsy and Behavior. Frontiers of Clinical Neurosciences (Vol 12.) New York: Wiley-Liss, 1991.

Dodrill CB, Breyer DN, Diamond MB, et al. Psychosocial problems among adults with epilepsy. Epilepsia 1984;25:168-175.

Hermann BP. The Relevance of Social Factors to Adjustment in Epilepsy. In O Devinsky, WH Theodore (eds), Epilepsy and Behavior. New York: Wiley-Liss, 1991;23-26.

Hermann BP, Vickrey B, Hays RD, et al. A comparison of health-related quality of life in patients with epilepsy, diabetes and multiple sclerosis. Epilepsy Res 1996;25:113-118.

Krumholtz A, Fisher RS, Lesser RP, et al. Driving and epilepsy: a review and reappraisal. JAMA 1991;265:622-626.

Lipman IJ, Lehman C. Consensus Conference on driver licensing and epilepsy: American Academy of Neurology, American Epilepsy Society, and Epilepsy Foundation of America. Epilepsia 1994;35:662-664.

Perrine KR. A new quality-of-life inventory for epilepsy patients: interim results. Epilepsia 1993;34(Suppl 4):S28-S33.

Salinsky MC, Wegener K, Sinnema F. Epilepsy driving laws and patient disclosure to physicians. Epilepsia 1992;33:469-472.
Smith DB, Treiman DM, Trimble MR (eds). Neurobehavioral Problems in Epilepsy. New York: Raven, 1990.
Spencer SS, Hunt PW. Quality of life in epilepsy. J Epilepsy 1996;9:3-13.
Taylor J, Chadwick D, Johnsons T. Risk of accidents in drivers with epilepsy. J Neurol Neurosurg Psychiatr 1996;60:621-627.
Treiman DM. Epilepsy and violence: medical and legal issues. Epilepsia 1986;27(Suppl 2): S77-S104.
Trimble MR, Dodson WE (eds). Epilepsy and Quality of Life. New York: Raven, 1994.

Suggested Reading

Aicardi J. Epilepsy in Children (2nd ed). New York: Raven, 1994.

Dam M, Lennart G (eds). Comprehensive Epileptology. New York: Raven, 1991.

Devinsky O (ed). Epilepsy 1: diagnosis and treatment. Neurol Clin 1993;11.

Devinsky O (ed). Epilepsy 2: special issues. Neurol Clin 1994;12.

Dodson WE, Pellock JM (eds). Pediatric Epilepsy: Diagnosis and Therapy. New York: Demos, 1993.

Duncan JS, Shorvon SD, Fish DR. Clinical Epilepsy. New York: Churchill Livingstone, 1995.

Engel J Jr. Seizures and Epilepsy. Philadelphia: F.A. Davis, 1989.

Engel J Jr, Pedley TA (eds). Epilepsy: A Comprehensive Textbook. New York: Lippincott-Raven, 1997.

French J. The long-term therapeutic management of epilepsy. Ann Intern Med 1994;120: 411-422.

Holmes GL. Epilepsy and Other Seizure Disorders. In BO Berg (ed), Principles of Child Neurology, New York: McGraw-Hill, 1996;223-284.

Jagoda A, Riggio S. Management of seizures in the emergency department. Emerg Med Clin North Am 1994;12:895-1139.

Jasper HH, Riggio S, Goldman-Rakic PS (eds). Epilepsy and the Functional Anatomy of the Frontal Lobe. Advances in Neurology (Vol 66). New York: Raven, 1995.

Levy RH, Mattson RH, Meldrum B (eds). Antiepileptic Drugs (4th ed). New York: Raven, 1995.

Malow BA. Sleep and epilepsy. Neurol Clin 1996;14:765-789.

Pedley TA, Meldrum BS (eds). Recent Advances in Epilepsy—6. New York: Churchill Livingstone 1995.

Penry JK, Daly DD (eds). Complex Partial Seizures and Their Treatment. Advances in Neurology (Vol 11). New York: Raven, 1975.

Porter RJ, Chadwick D (eds). The Epilepsies 2. Boston: Butterworth-Heinemann, 1997.

So EL. Update on epilepsy. Med Clin North Am 1993;77:203-214.

Wyllie E (ed). The Treatment of Epilepsy: Principles and Practice (2nd ed). Baltimore: Williams & Wilkins, 1997.

Appendix

Useful World Wide Web Sites for Professional and Lay Epilepsy Information

A wealth of scientific and practical information on epilepsy, in addition to many discussion groups and forums, is available on the Internet. The available information expands rapidly. Sites that the authors have found useful and that offer links to many other sites include the following:

- http://www.aesnet.org
  American Epilepsy Society home page.
- http://www.efa.org
  Epilepsy Foundation of America home page. Useful site for current information on driving regulations, legal issues, and epilepsy for patients and families; links.
- http://www.clae.ca
  Canadian League Against Epilepsy home page.
- http://www.epilepsy.ca
  Epilepsy Canada home page.
- http://www.epilepsyontario.org//index.html
  Epilepsy Ontario index of links.
- http://www.who.ch/ina/ngo/ngo088.htm
  International League Against Epilepsy home page.
- http://www.neuro.wustl.edu/epilepsy
  Site of the Washington University Comprehensive Epilepsy Program. One of the best starting points for information because of its extensive links.
- http://www.ttuhsc.edu/pages/neuro/ttep.htm
  Many useful links, including information on the ketogenic diet, epilepsy surgery, and pseudoseizures.
- http://www.epilepsy-international.com/english/issues/issmain.html
  Position papers on and discussions of various epilepsy issues, including driving, ketogenic diet, and legal aspects of epilepsy.
- http://www.ncbi.nlm.nih.gov/Omim/
  On-Line Mendelian Inheritance in Man. Excellent source on the latest genetic information on epilepsy and on genetic diseases that have epilepsy as a feature.

Index

Note: Page numbers followed by *f* indicate figures; page numbers followed by *t* indicate tables.